Gender Variant Children and Transgender Adolescents

Guest Editor

RICHARD R. PLEAK, MD

CHILD AND ADOLESCENT PSYCHIATRIC CLINICS OF NORTH AMERICA

www.childpsych.theclinics.com

Consulting Editor
HARSH K. TRIVEDI, MD

October 2011 • Volume 20 • Number 4

SAUNDERS an imprint of ELSEVIER, Inc.

W.B. SAUNDERS COMPANY
A Division of Elsevier Inc.

Elsevier Inc. • 1600 John F. Kennedy Boulevard • Suite 1800 • Philadelphia, Pennsylvania 19103-2899

http://www.childpsych.theclinics.com

CHILD AND ADOLESCENT PSYCHIATRIC CLINICS OF NORTH AMERICA Volume 20, Number 4
October 2011 ISSN 1056-4993, ISBN-13: 978-1-4557-1092-8

Editor: Sarah E. Barth

Child and Adolescent Psychiatric Clinics of North America (ISSN 1056-4993) is published quarterly by Elsevier Inc., 360 Park Avenue South, New York, NY 10010-1710. Months of issue are January, April, July, and October. Business and Editorial Offices: 1600 John F. Kennedy Boulevard, Suite 1800, Philadelphia, PA 19103-2899. Periodicals postage paid at New York, NY and additional mailing offices. Subscription prices are $275.00 per year (US individuals), $425.00 per year (US institutions), $139.00 per year (US students), $318.00 per year (Canadian individuals), $513.00 per year (Canadian institutions), $176.00 per year (Canadian students), $378.00 per year (international individuals), $513.00 per year (international institutions), and $176.00 per year (international students). International air speed delivery is included in all *Clinics* subscription prices. All prices are subject to change without notice. **POSTMASTER:** Send address changes to *Child and Adolescent Psychiatric Clinics of North America,* Elsevier Health Sciences Division, Subscription Customer Service, 3251 Riverport Lane, Maryland Heights, MO 63043. **Customer Service: 1-800-654-2452 (U.S. and Canada); 314-447-8871 (outside U.S. and Canada). Fax: 314-447-8029. E-mail: JournalsCustomerService-usa@ elsevier.com (for print support) or journalsonlinesupport-usa@elsevier.com (for online support).**

Reprints. For copies of 100 or more of articles in this publication, please contact the Commercial Reprints Department, Elsevier Inc., 360 Park Avenue South, New York, New York 10010-1710 Tel.: (212) 633-3812; Fax: (212) 462-1935, e-mail: reprints@elsevier.com.

Child and Adolescent Psychiatric Clinics of North America is covered in *MEDLINE/PubMed (Index Medicus), ISI, SSCI, Research Alert, Social Search, Current Contents,* and *EMBASE/Excerpta Medica.*

Printed and bound by CPI Group (UK) Ltd, Croydon, CR0 4YY

Transferred to Digital Print 2011

Contributors

CONSULTING EDITOR

HARSH K. TRIVEDI, MD
Associate Professor of Psychiatry, Vanderbilt University School of Medicine; and Executive Medical Director, and Chief of Staff, Vanderbilt Psychiatric Hospital, Nashville, Tennessee

CONSULTING EDITOR EMERITUS

ANDRÉS MARTIN, MD, MPH

FOUNDING CONSULTING EDITOR

MELVIN LEWIS, MBBS, FRCPSYCH, DCH

GUEST EDITOR

RICHARD R. PLEAK, MD
Associate Professor of Psychiatry, Director of Education in Child and Adolescent Psychiatry, Hofstra North Shore-LIJ School of Medicine; Zucker Hillside Hospital, Ambulatory Care Pavilion, Glen Oaks, New York; Associate Professor of Clinical Psychiatry and Behavioral Sciences, Albert Einstein College of Medicine; Chair, Sexual Orientation and Gender Identity Issues Committee, Bronx, New York; American Academy of Child & Adolescent Psychiatry

AUTHORS

STEWART L. ADELSON, MD
Assistant Clinical Professor, Division of Child and Adolescent Psychiatry, Columbia University College of Physicians and Surgeons; Adjunct Clinical Assistant Professor, Division of Child and Adolescent Psychiatry, Weill Medical College of Cornell University, New York, New York

PEGGY T. COHEN-KETTENIS, PhD
Professor of Medical Psychology, Department of Medical Psychology and Medical Social Work, VU University Medical Center, the Netherlands

ANNELOU L.C. DE VRIES, MD, PhD
Child and Adolescent Psychiatrist, Department of Child and Adolescent Psychiatry, VU University Medical Center, the Netherlands

WYLIE C. HEMBREE, MD
Department of Medicine, Division of Endocrinology, College of Physicians and Surgeons, Columbia University Medical Center, New York, New York

SARAH E. HERBERT, MD, MSW
Clinical Assistant Professor, Morehouse School of Medicine, Department of Psychiatry and Behavioral Sciences, Atlanta, Georgia

TONY KELSO, PhD
Associate Professor of Media Studies, Department of Mass Communication, Iona College, New Rochelle, New York

SCOTT F. LEIBOWITZ, MD
Instructor of Psychiatry, Department of Psychiatry, Children's Hospital Boston, Harvard Medical School, Boston, Massachusetts

EDGARDO J. MENVIELLE, MD, MSHS
Associate Professor of Psychiatry and Behavioral Sciences, George Washington University; Attending Psychiatrist, Department of Psychiatry, Children's National Medical Center, Washington, DC

HEINO F.L. MEYER-BAHLBURG, Dr rer nat
Professor of Clinical Psychology in Psychiatry, New York State Psychiatric Institute/Department of Psychiatry, Columbia University, New York, New York

RICHARD R. PLEAK, MD
Associate Professor of Psychiatry, Director of Education in Child and Adolescent Psychiatry, Hofstra North Shore-LIJ School of Medicine, Zucker Hillside Hospital, Ambulatory Care Pavilion, Glen Oaks, New York; Associate Professor of Clinical Psychiatry and Behavioral Sciences, Albert Einstein College of Medicine, Bronx, New York; Chair, Sexual Orientation and Gender Identity Issues Committee, American Academy of Child & Adolescent Psychiatry

D. TOWNSEND REINER, MA
Cambridge, Massachusetts

WILLIAM G. REINER, MD
Professor of Pediatric Urology, Departments of Urology and Psychiatry, Division of Child and Adolescent Psychiatry (Adjunct), University of Oklahoma Health Sciences Center, Oklahoma City, Oklahoma

LESLIE A. RODNAN, MD
Assistant Clinical Professor of Pediatrics, George Washington University, Washington, DC

SHANE SNOWDON
Center for LGBT Health and Equity, University of California, San Francisco, California

NORMAN P. SPACK, MD
Assistant Professor of Pediatrics, Division of Endocrinology, Children's Hospital Boston; Co-director, Gender Management Service, Children's Hospital Boston, Harvard Medical School, Boston, Massachusetts

THOMAS D. STEENSMA, MSc
Child Psychologist, Department of Medical Psychology and Medical Social Work, VU University Medical Center, the Netherlands

JOEL STODDARD, MD, MAS
Former: Department of Psychiatry and Behavioral Sciences, University of California, Davis, Health System, Sacramento, California; Current: Clinical Fellow, Section on Bipolar Spectrum Disorders, Emotion and Development Branch, National Institute of Mental Health, Bethesda, Maryland

HENDRY TON, MD, MS
Department of Psychiatry and Behavioral Sciences, University of California, Davis, Health System, Sacramento, California

CATHERINE TUERK, MA, APRN
Nurse Psychotherapist, Private Practice; Senior Consultant to the Gender and Sexuality Advocacy and Education Program, Children's National Medical Center, Washington, DC

DEBORAH L. WISNOWSKI
Co-Founder Stepping Stones Support Group; Board Member, Parents, Families, and Friends of Lesbians and Gays, New York City Families of Color and Allies (PFLAG FCA NYC), New York, New York

HAYLEY WOOD, PhD
Gender Identity Service, Child, Youth, and Family Program, Centre for Addiction and Mental Health, Toronto, Ontario, Canada

KENNETH J. ZUCKER, PhD
Head, Gender Identity Service, Child, Youth, and Family Program, Centre for Addiction and Mental Health; Psychologist-in-Chief, Centre for Addiction and Mental Health; Professor, Department of Psychiatry, University of Toronto, Toronto, Ontario, Canada; Chair, DSM-5 Sexual and Gender Identity Disorders Work Group

Contents

> An expanding number of mental health professionals evaluate, advocate for, treat, and refer gender variant children and transgender youth. Official recognition of these persons and their needs as well as support for improvement and change come from several different national surveys and professional policy and accreditation organizations. Being informed about these and other available resources can help with patient advocacy. The author provides a reading list for youth and families, definitions of terms, a history of youth gender variance, history and policies of professional organizations, and recent reports and initiatives. An appendix with a patient's first-hand story is included.

> Children with disorders of sex development have similarities to, but also marked contrasts with, children with normal anatomy but who have gender dysphoria. Understanding gender identity development in children with sex disorders will probably help us understand typical gender identity development more than in understanding gender development in children with gender identity disorder.

> Individuals born with a somatic disorder of sex development (DSD) have high rates of gender-atypical behavior, gender uncertainty, gender

evaluation and what treatments and other resources are available for them and their families. Where there seem to be differences between boys and girls with gender identity issues, they will be noted.

Peggy T. Cohen-Kettenis, Thomas D. Steensma, and Annelou L.C. de Vries

In the Netherlands, gender dysphoric adolescents may be eligible for puberty suppression at age 12, subsequent cross-sex hormone treatment at age 16, and gender reassignment surgery at age 18. Initially, a thorough assessment is made of the gender dysphoria and vulnerabilities in functioning or circumstances. Psychological interventions and/or gender reassignment may be offered. Psychological interventions are offered if the adolescent needs to explore gender identity and treatment wishes, suffers from coexisting problems, or needs support and counseling during gender reassignment. Although more studies are necessary, this approach seems to contribute significantly to the well-being of gender dysphoric adolescents.

Scott F. Leibowitz and Norman P. Spack

Few interdisciplinary treatment programs that tend to the needs of youth with gender nonconforming behaviors, expressions, and identities exist in academic medical centers with formal residency training programs. Despite this, the literature provides evidence that these youth have higher rates of poor psychosocial adjustment and suicide attempts. This article explores the logistical considerations involved in developing a specialized interdisciplinary service to these gender minority youth in accordance with the existing treatment guidelines. Demographic data will be presented and treatment issues will be explored. The impact that a specialized interdisciplinary treatment program has on clinical expansion, research development, education and training, and community outreach initiatives is discussed.

Wylie C. Hembree

Pubertal suppression at Tanner stage 2 should be considered in adolescents with persistent gender identity disorder (GID). Issues related to achievement of adult height, timing of initiating sex steroid treatment, future fertility options, preventing uterine bleeding, and required modifications of genital surgery remain concerns. Concerns have been raised about altering neuropsychological development during cessation of puberty and reinitiation of puberty by the sex steroid opposite those determined by genetic sex. Collaborative assessment and treatment of dysphoric adolescents with persistent GID resolves these concerns and deepens our understanding of gender development.

Therapy for transgender, transsexual, and gender variant persons has traditionally assisted individuals in the process of adjusting to their newly adopted gender role. Increasingly, younger gender variant patients, teens and preteens, present to the clinical consultation raising the need to develop therapeutic interventions that better address the psychosocial needs of minors. The Gender and Sexuality Development Program at Children's National Medical Center (CNMC) in Washington, DC (http://www.childrensnational.org/gendervariance), provides outpatient psychosocial evaluations and therapeutic services for children, adolescents, and their families.

This article is a first-person account of a father's journey to lovingly accept his young gender variant son, who began to show traits and preferences more common to girls almost from birth. The dad's efforts to discover constructive parenting strategies for raising his boy are also detailed. Experiences described begin with guilt and awareness of his own difficulty in coming to terms with his son's behavior, progress toward seeking and finding support and guidance, and eventually learning to embrace his son as he is, perhaps with questions about his own liberality and apprehensions about his boy's future.

This article overviews the challenges parents face raising gender non-conforming children. The author is the mother of a fifteen year old gender non-conforming (GNC) child and co-founder of Stepping Stones Support Group which organizes support programs for families of GNC. The article discusses social challenges, educational challenges and internal conflicts the author has experienced while raising her child. The author also discusses the process of founding Stepping Stones and the importance having support has played in her and her child's life.

The media and the public's reaction have created the impression that gender variant behaviors of many children are indicative of later transsexual identities. This has suggested to some parents that the best way to manage their sons' gender variance and perhaps gender dysphoria is to allow them to dress as girls in increasingly more situations. For some this becomes a transition to living full-time as a girl. However, the author believes that most of these boys would be better served by helping them develop an awareness of the many ways of being a boy, stigma-reducing social strategies, and facilitating a positive gay identity.

Gender minority children and adolescents present to a wide variety of health professionals for gender-related care and other care. However, few professionals may be prepared to meet their needs. Unprepared clinicians risk developing insufficient therapeutic rapport, missing salient information, and inadvertently contributing to risk. In this article the authors outline ways to address these gaps at all training levels to meet the needs of gender minority children and adolescents. They provide practical resources for colleagues interested in expanding education opportunities in their own community. In the end, competency in gender minority health should improve access to care for these youths.

FORTHCOMING ISSUES

RECENT ISSUES

THE CLINICS ARE NOW AVAILABLE ONLINE!

Access your subscription at:
www.theclinics.com

Foreword
Finding Clarity Through the Confusion

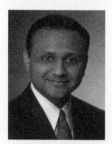

Harsh K. Trivedi, MD
Consulting Editor

Childhood and adolescence are times of unparalleled personal development and growth. From the child that takes his first steps to the young adult that embarks for college, there are many milestones and great achievements along the way. The process of "growing-up" is marked by many points of confusion. From figuring out how to put one foot in front of the other; to figuring out who you are and how you fit in with your family, your peer group, and your community—there are many questions and concerns that we all need to deal with. It is this path toward adulthood that I think of as the path of finding clarity through confusion. Important ingredients in this process include exploring the world around you, being inquisitive, and discovering the truth.

The impetus for requesting that Dr Pleak develop an issue on gender-variant children and transgender adolescents derives from a practical clinical need. While caring for youth on our inpatient psychiatry service at Vanderbilt Psychiatric Hospital, I am keenly aware of the need to truly understand my patients and their concerns. As I get to know my patients, I am also keenly aware of where my own knowledge-base and clinical skills fail me. How do I appropriately evaluate gender-variant and transgender youth? How do I help my patients appropriately deal with their questions and concerns? What do I say to parents and guardians as they ask me (the "expert") on how to help their child? As I develop a treatment plan, how do I meaningfully address issues related to youth who are gender variant or are transgendered?

As this is a quickly developing field and few authoritative (and up-to-date) resources exist, the need for this issue is clear. I want to sincerely thank Richard Pleak for compiling many of the world's experts for this issue. I am also grateful to each of our authors for sharing their expertise on this topic. As we each find clarity through the confusion in our quest for knowledge and lifelong learning, let us hope that we can

Child Adolesc Psychiatric Clin N Am 20 (2011) xiii–xv
doi:10.1016/j.chc.2011.08.015
1056-4993/11/$ – see front matter © 2011 Elsevier Inc. All rights reserved.

childpsych.theclinics.com

better aid our patients as they grow up and progress down the path of finding their own truths.

Harsh K. Trivedi, MD
Vanderbilt Psychiatric Hospital
1601 23rd Avenue South, Suite 1157
Nashville, TN 37212, USA

E-mail address:
harsh.k.trivedi@vanderbilt.edu

Preface

Gender-Variant Children and Transgender Adolescents

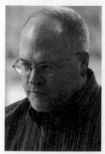

Richard R. Pleak, MD
Guest Editor

This issue is the third since the beginning of the *Child and Adolescents Psychiatric Clinics of North America* in 1992 to deal substantially with gender identity issues in youth. The first was Volume 2(3), Sexual and Gender Identity Disorders, in 1993; the second was Volume 13(3), Sex and Gender, in 2004. Two authors in the Volume 2, 1993 issue are contributors here: Drs Zucker and Meyer-Bahlburg; two authors in the Volume 13, 2004 issue are contributors here: Drs Zucker and Reiner. This issue differs from the others in being exclusively about gender identity issues: gender variance and transgenderism. The consulting *Clinics* editor, Dr Harsh Trivedi, identified a need for this issue in light of recent developments in the field and the increasing numbers of mental health clinicians requesting more information pertaining to these youth.

Variations in behavior and personal identity are hallmarks of the human race. When those variations are to a degree considered by society out of proportion to a perceived normality or to an extreme that may cause harm to the individual or society, the variation is generally regarded as objectionable, abnormal, or pathological. The concept of what is male or female in most societies today is ingrained in culture largely as dichotomous, male vs female, "Mars" vs "Venus," one or the other, opposite sexes. Individual variations in maleness or femaleness in behavior and identity, therefore, challenge this dichotomy and become troublesome for other individuals and for society. Over time, such challenges may become gradually more commonplace, accepted, and eventually normal for a given society. Consider the oft-referenced example of homosexuality, listed as a psychiatric disorder in Diagnostic and Statistical Manual for Mental Disorders until 1973[1] and seen as challenging conventional opposite-sex eroticism. Since the 1973 depathologizing of homosexuality and since homosexual civil rights events such as Stonewall in 1969, gays and lesbians have been more open and visible, and homosexuality has slowly become more accepted as normal by society. As another example, consider women entering

Child Adolesc Psychiatric Clin N Am 20 (2011) xv–xx
doi:10.1016/j.chc.2011.08.007
1056-4993/11/$ – see front matter
childpsych.theclinics.com

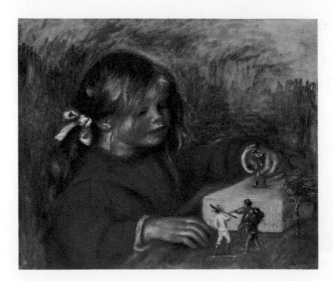

Fig. 1

medicine in the United States. It was regarded as highly unusual and objectionable (although not pathological) in the 19th and much of the 20th century for women to enter medical school, as Gertrude Stein did in 1897. However, it is now not only commonplace, but women in medical school reached parity with men in 2003. Examples in clothing, jewelry, and hair abound: pants in women, earrings in men, long hair/short hair.

Two paintings from the 19th to early 20th centuries are illustrative of changes in gender norms over time. I often show the painting in **Fig. 1** to my residents and fellows in the context of our didactics on gender variance in normal development seminars. After discussing aspects of cross-gender behavior in children, I ask them to identify the painter and to give their impression of the painting. After figuring out that the painter is Renoir, most trainees will say something like, "it's a little girl playing with cowboys and Indians, so she's engaged in cross-gender play." I then identify the title as *Claude Renoir at Play*, from 1905, a painting of Renoir's youngest *son* at age 4 years, from the Musée de l'Orangerie in Paris. My trainees are frequently surprised that pink was the norm for boys in Europe in those times, the same for long hair with bows, and how radically this changed in the 20th century. I do the same with another portrait, that shown in **Fig. 2**, *Young Boy with a Whip*, by an unknown American painter in about 1840, from the Honolulu Academy of Arts. Most trainees think that this is a painting of a boy cross-dressed as a girl; however, the boy's frilly pink dress and ribbon-bowed shoes are gender-typical for his time, but would be considered extremely gender-atypical now.

Despite acceptance over time of some variations in maleness or femaleness, many others remain more rigidly dichotomous. This is generally more so for what are seen as normal male behaviors by most societies. While acceptable and normal for girls to wear pants, it is still regarded as abnormal and pathological for boys to wear skirts and dresses or make-up (see also my section on history in this issue). Substantial and unusual variation in maleness or femaleness in behavior or identity is generally designated as cross-gender, gender-variant, gender-atypical, or transgender. Children and adolescents manifesting such variation are often considered to be abnormal and therefore referred for evaluation and treatment to mental health professionals. Should this variation be

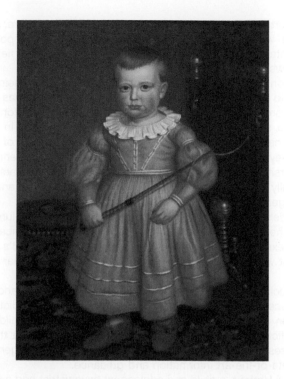

Fig. 2

substantial enough, the child or adolescent would meet criteria in DSM-IV[2] for gender identity disorder (GID) or in DSM-5 (www.dsm5.org) for gender dysphoria.

Cross-gender behavior and identity are at not all new phenomena, but they have been considered to be rare, especially in youth; for this reason, the majority of mental health professionals have had very limited experience with or training about these youth[3] (see the article by Stoddard and coworkers in this issue for remedies for this). In the last two to three decades, more and more cross-gender youth have been coming to the attention of mental health professionals. This can be regarded in part as an increased openness of cross-gender youth to disclose, heightened awareness of cross-gender behavior and identity in parents and others, and/or a genuine increase in youth with cross-gender behavior and identity.

The number of child psychiatrists who have significant experience working with cross-gender youth is very limited; at present, fewer than a dozen exist in North America, with a somewhat higher number of psychologists. Barriers to cross-gender behavior and identity in youth are uncommon, most training programs have little in their curricula or clinical experiences with these youth, and because these variations can be very challenging and uncomfortable for the individual provider acculturated in the dichotomy of maleness/femaleness. This issue of the *Clinics* is an effort to decrease these barriers and help mental health professionals gain more knowledge of and interest in working with cross-gender youth.

THIS ISSUE'S CONTRIBUTIONS

Given the paucity of expert clinicians in the area of gender variance and transgenderism in children and adolescents, this issue of the *Clinics* represents a very substantial proportion of the field: most of the major players are here. After my review of terminologies with clinical examples, historical information, policies of major professional mental health organizations, and advancements in the field, a plethora of information follows in the other articles by these experts.

Two articles on intersex children are included. Dr William Reiner, a pediatric urologist and child psychiatrist at the University of Oklahoma who has done important research on disorders of sexual development and has cared for many intersex children, and his son Townsend Reiner review gender identity in the context of intersex conditions, providing an erudite in-depth understanding of these complex issues. Heino Meyer-Bahlburg, a psychologist and psychoneuroendocrinologist at Columbia University and a pioneering expert in the fields of intersex and gender variance, carefully considers the issues of monitoring gender and questions of reassigning the gender of intersex children.

Dr Stewart Adelson, a child and adolescent psychiatrist at Columbia University, adroitly details the long and complex process of developing clinical guidelines for lesbian, gay, bisexual, and transgender (LGBT) youth, giving a bird's eye view of the proceedings that will be of assistance to others engaged in similar efforts in other organizations.

Dr Kenneth Zucker, a psychologist at the University of Toronto and director of the child and adolescent gender identity clinic at their Centre for Addiction and Mental Health, has been a leading researcher in gender variance in children for several decades. His article with Dr Haley Woods, also a psychologist at the University of Toronto, discusses the critical evaluation procedure to ascertain gender variance in children with state-of-the-art information and guidance.

Dr Sarah (Sally) Herbert, a child and adolescent psychiatrist and a social worker at Morehouse School of Medicine in Atlanta and an expert on girls with gender variance and transgender boys, provides an important discussion of gender identity issues in children born as female, a topic covered much less often than that of natal boys with gender variance.

Dr Peggy Cohen-Kettenis is a psychologist and pioneer in the research and treatment of transgender adolescents in the Netherlands. Her colleagues at the Free University in Amsterdam, Dr Thomas Steensma, a psychologist, and Dr Annelou de Vries, a child and adolescent psychiatrist and psychologist, richly describe their seminal clinic for transgender adolescents, which has been a model worldwide for their very careful screening, evaluation, and follow-up of patients for possible puberty suspension and sex reassignment.

The Amsterdam clinic has served as a model for the founding of a similar clinic at Boston Children's Hospital, one of the few such in the United States. The development of this clinic is the subject of the article by Drs Scott Leibowitz and Norman Spack. Dr Leibowitz is an early career child and adolescent psychiatrist at Harvard who has quickly become one of the new experts in the area; Dr Spack is a pediatric endocrinologist and one of a very few in the United States who treat transgender adolescents, another pioneer in the field.

Dr Wylie Hembree is an endocrinologist affiliated with Columbia University and is also one of a very few endocrinologists in the United States who treat transgender adolescents and is active in international professional organizations advocating for transgender health. His article reviews the guidelines he and Drs Spack and Cohen-Kettenis were instrumental in developing for the Endocrine Society for pubertal suspension and hormonal treatment of transgender adolescents.[4]

Dr Edgardo Menvielle, a child and adolescent psychiatrist at Children's National Medical Center and George Washington University in Washington, DC, is a pioneer in developing services, including support groups and listserves, for parents and their gender-variant children. His article with Dr Leslie Rodnan, a pediatrician also at George Washington University, provides information about these groups and their crucial help for parents.

We are very fortunate that two parents of gender-variant children have contributed articles about their experiences dealing with gender issues. Dr Kelso aptly addresses the conflicts and concerns that are almost universal for the parents. Ms Wisnowski discusses how her gender-variant child, who is now undergoing puberty suspension, stimulated her to organize a greatly needed support group for parents, the first in the New York City area since the groups that Dr Dennis Anderson and I led in 1991–1994 at Long Island Jewish Medical Center.[5]

Catherine Tuerk, a nurse in private practice in Washington, DC, was a cofounder with Dr Menvielle of the groups for parents and their gender-variant children at Children's National Medical Center. Her article speaks as a parent of a gender-variant child who is also a clinician in the field and discusses concerns parents have as well as questions about excessively early gender reassignment of prepubertal children, a controversial subject.

Dr Joel Stoddard is a research fellow in child and adolescent psychiatry at the National Institute of Mental Health in Bethesda, MD and was formerly at the University of California, Davis; he has already been very active in working on gender issues in youth as a trainee. Dr Scott Leibowitz, profiled above, Dr Hendry Ton, a psychiatrist at the University of California, Davis, and Shane Snowdon, Director of the Center for LGBT Health and Equity, University of California, San Francisco, join Dr Stoddard in the final article, summarizing how medical education can be improved to foster better care for LGBT youth. Their recommendations and resources are exceptionally helpful in planning for education and training on these often-neglected areas.

BREAKING DEVELOPMENTS REGARDING GENDER IDENTITY IN YOUTH

As this *Clinics* issue goes to press, there are new developments in progress that will have bearing on this *Clinics* issue's contents and are referenced in most of the articles here. These include the following:

○ DSM-5. The DSM-IV[2] is in revision, with DSM-5 due for publication in 2013. At the time of this writing, the DSM-IV diagnosis of gender identity disorder will be revised to be gender dysphoria in children and gender dysphoria in adolescents and adults, with changes in the criteria for the diagnosis (see www.dsm5.org). Gender identity disorder, not otherwise specified (NOS), is to become unspecified gender identity disorder, in line with changing "NOS" designations to "unspecified." The gender dysphoria diagnoses will be in a separate section rather than part of what was titled "Sexual and Gender Identity Disorders" in DSM-IV. The DSM-5 Sexual and Gender Identity Disorders Work Group includes three contributors to this issue: Drs Zucker (chair), Meyer-Bahlburg, and Cohen-Kettenis.

○ American Academy of Child and Adolescent Psychiatry (AACAP) Practice Parameters. Dr Adelson's article in this issue details the background and developmental process for psychiatry's first practice guidelines on gender identity and sexual orientation issues, by the AACAP. These Practice Parameters are due for review by AACAP's Executive Council, with potential for publication in 2012.

○ American Psychiatric Association (APA) Practice Guidelines. The APA initiated a Task Force on GID several years ago, chaired by William Byne, MD, PhD, to advise the APA's Board of Trustees as to whether or not the evidence base supports development of Practice Guidelines on GID by the APA. The Task

Force's report recommended that such Guidelines should be developed; its report with recommendations is under review by the Board of Trustees. Three authors in this *Clinics* issue are members of this Task Force on GID: Drs Meyer-Bahlburg, Menvielle, and Pleak.

A PERSONAL NOTE

Editing this *Clinics* issue has been a pleasure, with such superb and accomplished authors whom I deeply thank, but it has also been daunting, given the rapidly evolving landscape in the realm of gender identity. Major advancements are on the horizon; some changes, such as diagnostic terminology and treatment guidelines, will be evident and resolved as this issue goes to press. The reader's challenge is to incorporate these new developments into what is learned here; this issue is a snapshot in time of a target quickly moving along the road toward greatly improved knowledge and patient care.

Richard R. Pleak, MD
Hofstra North Shore-LIJ School of Medicine
Albert Einstein College of Medicine
Zucker Hillside Hospital, Ambulatory Care Pavilion
75-59 263rd Street
Glen Oaks, NY 11004, USA

E-mail address:
rpleak@nshs.edu

REFERENCES

1. Bayer R. Homosexuality and American Psychiatry. Princeton, NJ: Princeton University Press; 1987.
2. APA (American Psychiatric Association). Diagnostic and statistical manual of mental disorders, 4th Edition (Text Revision). Washington, DC: American Psychiatric Association; 2000.
3. Townsend MH, Wallick MM, Pleak RR, et al. Gay and lesbian issues in child and adolescent psychiatry training as reported by training directors. J Am Acad Child Adoles Psychiatry 1997;36(6):764–8.
4. Hembree WC, Cohen-Kettenis PT, Delemarre-van de Waal HA, et al. Endocrine treatment of transsexual persons: an Endocrine Society clinical practice guideline. J Clin Endocrinol Metab 2009;94(9):3132–54.
5. Pleak RR, Anderson DA. A parents group for boys with gender identity disorders. Paper presented at Harry Benjamin International Gender Dysphoria Association Biennial Conference, XIII International Symposium, New York, NY; 1993.

Dedications

To past and current mental health pioneers in helping gender-variant children and transgender adolescents, to the growing number of new experts joining us in this exciting and important area, to the memory of the deceased pioneers Dennis Anderson and Bill Stone, to a fellow traveler, Karen Wellen, and to my (legal) husband, Jon W. Weatherman.

Richard R. Pleak, MD

Hofstra North Shore-LIJ School of Medicine
Albert Einstein College of Medicine
Zucker Hillside Hospital, Ambulatory Care Pavilion
75-59 263rd Street
Glen Oaks, NY 11004, USA

E-mail address:
rpleak@nshs.edu

Child Adolesc Psychiatric Clin N Am 20 (2011) xxi
doi:10.1016/j.chc.2011.08.016
1056-4993/11/$ – see front matter © 2011 Elsevier Inc. All rights reserved.

Gender Identity Issues in Youth: Opportunities, Terminologies, Histories, and Advancements

Richard R. Pleak, MD[a,b,c],*

KEYWORDS

• Gender identity • Gender variance • Transgender • Child
• Adolescent

This *Clinics* issue comes at a propitious and opportune time. An expanding number of mental health professionals will have the opportunity to evaluate, advocate for, and provide treatment and referrals for gender variant children and transgender youth in the coming years, as parents and society in general recognize and acknowledge cross-gender behavior and identity in youth. Official recognition for this need and support for improvement and change comes from several different national surveys and professional policy and accreditation organizations. This information is exceedingly helpful in our advocacy for the best care for our patients.

The general public is becoming more and more aware of gender variance and transgenderism in youth by the sharing of information on the Internet; by the growing numbers of people disclosing their transgender identities, especially celebrities such as Chaz (formerly Chastity) Bono,[1] Renée Richards,[2] Alexis Arquette, and public figures such as politicians; by increased news reports, for example, Kids Challenge Gender Identity Earlier—And Get Support, *Seattle Times*, July 30, 2011,[3] and Boys Will Be Boys? Not in These Families, *New York Times*, June 10, 2011[4]; by antibullying initiatives such as the It Gets Better *YouTube* campaign; by outreach efforts of lesbian, gay, bisexual, and transgender (LGBT) organizations such as the Gender Identity Project of New York City's LGBT Center (www.gaycenter.org/gip); by heightened awareness of specific clinical programs (eg, the articles in this issue by Menvielle and Rodnan; Cohen-Kettenis, Steensma, and de Vries; and Leibowitz and

The author has nothing to disclose.
[a] Hofstra North Shore-LIJ School of Medicine, Glen Oaks, NY, USA
[b] Albert Einstein College of Medicine, Glen Oaks, NY, USA
[c] Sexual Orientation and Gender Identity Issues Committee, Glen Oaks, NY, USA
* Corresponding author. Zucker Hillside Hospital, Ambulatory Care Pavilion, 75-59 263rd Street, Glen Oaks, NY 11004, USA.
E-mail address: rpleak@nshs.edu

Child Adolesc Psychiatric Clin N Am 20 (2011) 601–625
doi:10.1016/j.chc.2011.08.006
1056-4993/11/$ – see front matter © 2011 Elsevier Inc. All rights reserved.

Spack); and by the small but rapidly increasing literature for youth and families specifically about gender identity.

A selected list of such books from 1985 to the present follows in order of publication date. The number of books has increased exponentially since the start of the 21st century.

William's Doll, by Charlotte Zolotow and William Pene Du Bois, 1985[5]

Is He A Girl?, by Louis Sachar and Barbara Sullivan, 1993[6]

Always My Child: A Parent's Guide to Understanding Your Gay, Lesbian, Bisexual, Transgender, or Questioning Son or Daughter, Kevin Jennings and Pat Shapiro, 2002[7]

Trans Forming Families: Real Stories About Transgendered Loved Ones, 2nd Edition, by Jessica Xavier, Mary Boenke, and Arlene Istar Lev, 2003[8]

Luna, by Julie Anne Peters, 2006[9]

Gender Identity: The Ultimate Teen Guide, by Cynthia Winfield, 2006[10]

Mom, I Need to Be a Girl, by Just Evelyn, 2007[11]

Dude, You're a Fag: Masculinity and Sexuality in High School, by C. J. Pascoe, 2007[12]

Transparent: Love, Family, and Living the T with Transgender Teens, by Cris Beam, 2008[13]

The Transgender Child: A Handbook for Families and Professionals, by Stephanie Brill and Rachel Pepper, 2008[14]

10,000 Dresses, by Marcus Ewert and Rex Ray, 2008[15]

The Queer Child, or Growing Sideways in the Twentieth Century, by Kathryn Bond Stockton, 2009[16]

Be Who You Are, by Jennifer Carr and Bea Rumback, 2010[17]

My Princess Boy, by Cheryl Kilodavis and Suzanne DeSimone, 2010[18]

Youth with Gender Issues: Seeking an Identity, by Kenneth McIntosh and Ida Walker, 2010[19]

Teens: Being Gay, Lesbian, Bisexual, or Transgender: GLBT Teens and Society, by Jeanne Nagle, 2010[20]

Teens: Being Gay, Lesbian, Bisexual, or Transgender: Home and Family Relationships, by Tamra Orr, 2010[21]

Teens: Being Gay, Lesbian, Bisexual, or Transgender: Friendship, Dating, and Relationships, by Simone Payment, 2010[22]

Teens: Being Gay, Lesbian, Bisexual, or Transgender: Life at School and the Community, by Richard Worth, 2010[23]

Feeling Wrong in Your Own Body: Understanding What It Means to Be Transgender, by Jaime Seba, 2010[24]

I am mJ, by Cris Beam, 2011[25]

Gender Born, Gender Made: Raising Healthy Gender-Nonconforming Children, by Diane Ehrensaft, 2011[26]

Helping Your Transgender Teen: A Guide for Parents, by Irwin Krieger, 2011[27]

GLBTQ: The Survival Guide for Gay, Lesbian, Bisexual, Transgender, and Questioning Teens, by Kelly Huegel, 2011[28]

All I Want To Be Is Me, by Phyllis Rothblatt, 2011[29]

It Gets Better: Coming Out, Overcoming Bullying, and Creating a Life Worth Living, by Dan Savage and Terry Miller, 2011[30]

GENDER TERMINOLOGY, WITH EXAMPLES AND REFLECTIONS

Terms used to describe gender variant or transgender youth vary greatly from person to person. Most of the authors in this *Clinics* issue define such terms themselves. Here, the author gives suggested definitions with some examples as he, his colleagues, and his patients use these terms. When working with patients and families or associates and trainees who use gender and sex terms to describe themselves or others, a key competence is to not assume the meaning is the same to you as it is to them, but rather to ask others how the terms apply to or for them. With teenagers in particular, use of these terms and the meanings they hold may shift repeatedly over time, so a continuous dialogue regarding the person's description of his/her gender identity is crucial. The "proper" terminology is that which the patient uses.

Sex, gender—These terms are often used interchangeably; however, sex is usually considered the biological origins and aspects of maleness/femaleness, whereas gender is considered more the social construct of what a society, culture, family, or peers consider maleness/femaleness. Male or female sex includes sexually dimorphic anatomy (eg, penis, breasts, parts of the brain) and physiology (eg, different ratios of certain hormones); sex is essentially constant, evolving over long periods of time. Gender includes what a society or system considers typical for males or females at a certain time or situation (eg, clothing, hair, professions, toys); gender is more fluid, rapidly changeable over time and circumstance: gender is not what it was.

Gender identity, gender role—Gender identity is a person's inner or personal sense of whether s/he is male or female, or how male, female, or in-between male and female s/he feels. Young children, especially in the stage of preoperational thinking, may believe this gender role is something that can be very transient and changing, whereas older children, teens, and adults feel gender identity is more permanent. Because the sense of one's maleness/femaleness is so certain and unquestioned by the majority of people, most have tremendous difficulty understanding this feeling in others, especially in the absence of observable differences. The person may not disclose his/her gender identity to others; parents (and therapists) are often perplexed trying to figure out the child's "true" gender identity because his/her behavior may not reveal gender identity. Gender role is the outward manifestation of maleness/femaleness in behaviors, speech, clothing, toy and game preferences, role-playing, fantasies, peer selection, interests, and so on. As such, gender role is more of a controllable, or adaptable, characteristic, which may or may not be congruent with the person's gender identity.

Cross-gender, gender variant, gender atypical, gender nonconformity—For the purposes of this article, these terms as seen as equivalent and connote behaviors and/or identities that are outside what is considered normal or typical by a society or culture for an individual's natal sex or assigned gender as male or female. Girls with cross-gender behavior are often called tomboys, which is to an extent considered a normal variation in most Western societies, whereas boys with cross-gender behavior are often called sissies, which is generally seen with derogation and the behavior or identity is seen as abnormal. *Gender variant* is the term that has become more commonly used in the past decade. *Gender-referred* and *gender disturbed* were terms used in the older literature for children referred to mental health professionals because of gender variance, particularly before a disorder of gender identity was categorized in American psychiatry[31] (see following discussion).

Transgender—An umbrella term applied primarily to adolescents or adults who have a cross-gender identity varying from a small degree to completely opposite their natal, or birth, sex to male or female. Most users include transsexuals under the larger transgender umbrella, whereas others do not. Many professionals hesitate to use this term to describe prepubertal cross-gender children because of the outcome of the majority of these children not being transgender in adolescence or adulthood. (For a discussion of this topic, see articles in this issue by Adelson; Herbert; Cohen-Kettenis Steensma, and de Vries; Leibowitz and Spack; Hembree; and Menvielle and Rodnan.)

However, one finds descriptors of transgender children by some authors such as Brill and Pepper.[14]

Trans—Often used as a shorthand form of transgender or transsexual; *tranny* is an informal slang term used by some trans people to refer to themselves or other trans people and often is used by nontrans people as a pejorative. *Transboy* or *transgender boy* refers to a natal girl who is becoming or has become a boy; *transgirl* or *transgender girl* refers to a natal boy who is becoming or has become a girl.

Transsexual—A term applied primarily to adolescents or adults who have a cross-gender identity completely opposite their natal or assigned sex of either male or female and who wish to, are in the process of, or have completed transition from one sex to the other with hormones and/or surgery. Some would not use the term *transsexual* for a person who has completed transition, instead using *man* or *woman* for description; some use the term *transman* or *transwoman* to describe the person as the sex s/he has become. The descriptor *MTF* designates male-to-female and *FTM* female-to-male. The proposed diagnosis in the *Diagnostic and Statistical Manual of Mental Disorders, 5th Edition* (DSM-5) of gender dysphoria in adolescents or adults includes the specifier *post-transition* to indicate the individual who "has transitioned to full-time living in the desired gender (with or without legalization of gender change) and has undergone (or is undergoing) at least one cross-sex medical procedure or treatment regimen,"[32] thereby maintaining a psychiatric diagnosis for a person whose gender identity is now consistent with the (new) biologic/anatomic sex although not with the natal sex: this proposal has come under considerable criticism. *Transsexualism* was a diagnostic term in DSM-III[33] and DSM-III-R[34]; the term was changed to *gender identity disorder* in DSM-IV[35] but remains a diagnostic term in the *International Statistical Classification of Diseases and Related Health Problems, 10th Revision.*[36]

Cisgender—Gender identity/behavior consistent with the natal, or birth, sex, as opposed to *trans*gender. Not commonly used.

Gender identity disorder of childhood (GIDC) or *gender identity disorder of adolescence or adulthood, nontranssexual type (GIDAANT)*—GIDC was a diagnosis in the 1980 DSM-III,[33] and both GIDC and GIDAANT were diagnoses in the 1987 DSM-III-R.[34] Before DSM-III in 1980, there were no gender identity diagnoses in DSM; pre-DSM-III, children and adolescents with gender variance referred to clinicians were primarily described in the literature as gender-referred. DSM-III's GIDC, GIDAANT, and transsexualism diagnoses were lumped into one diagnosis, gender identity disorder, in 1994's DSM-IV.[35] In DSM-5, gender identity disorder is proposed to be split into three categories: gender dysphoria in children, gender dysphoria in adolescents or adults, and unspecified gender dysphoria.[32] Ethical and practical issues of using the DSM gender identity diagnoses are addressed elsewhere in this issue and have been addressed over the past several decades by several investigators.[eg,37–39]

Gender incongruence—This term was an early proposed diagnostic term (2009–2011) in the development of DSM-5 for the revision of the DSM-IV diagnosis of gender identity disorder. As a rarely used term, *gender incongruence* had an advantage of not being laden with a previous history of varying use and controversy and possibly being less stigmatizing; it was undesirable to some because of its paucity of previous use. This proposal was revised to the currently proposed diagnostic label of gender dysphoria in early 2011.

Gender dysphoria—This term describes the inner sense of distress with one's assigned gender, often resulting in impairment in functioning or social relationships such as those with family members or in school. The term has been used for decades[40] for youth and adults with gender variance. Many gender variant children or transgender youth do not express or experience distress/dysfunction with their assigned gender—although they may desire to be the other sex—even if their families or others become distressed. The proposed DSM-5 diagnostic terms for the revised DSM-IV diagnosis of gender identity disorder are *gender dysphoria in children* and *gender dysphoria in adolescents or adults*, with the dysphoria criterion being clinically significant distress or impairment or a significantly increased risk of suffering.[32] How this "risk of suffering" is to be ascertained or quantified may be delineated by the time of DSM-5's publication in 2013.

Assigned gender—This term indicates the gender of rearing assigned to a child by the parents or guardians; most often it is the same as the natal sex, but it may not be for some children with disorders of sexual development (intersex) and very rarely for nonintersex children.

Genderqueer—This lay term is commonly used to indicate a gender identity in-between the poles of male or female or outside of this spectrum. Some other lay terms that have been used to indicate various states of nonmale/nonfemale identity are *third gender, third sex, bigender, on the spectrum, in-between, androgyne, gender outlaw, multigender, genderless, agender*, and *pangender*. Such terms and other newly coined terms are often used by younger people trying to define themselves differently from what they see as insufficient or inadequate descriptors in the literature, on the Internet, or from their elders.

Genderfluid—Indicates that the person feels fluid or flexible within the spectrum of male to female; this may change from day to day or over years. Gender fluidity and sexual fluidity are considered to be found more often in natal females.[41]

Gender spectrum or ***gender continuum***—Indicates identity from female to male and all degrees in between. A simple conceptualization may be shown as follows:

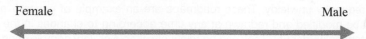

This gender identity spectrum or "thermometer" can be especially useful when working with people whose cognitive development is not (yet) in abstract reasoning or formal operations, in other words those in concrete operations or preoperational thinking such as children, preteens, many young adolescents, and those with developmental delays including autism spectrum disorders. Children and adolescents can chart their current identity and/or their desired identity along this spectrum; the designation can be for identity and/or behavior, such as how they appear to others (perceived gender). The author often has the person indicate these aspects with vertical marks with the date and which identity the mark represents entered above or below the mark.

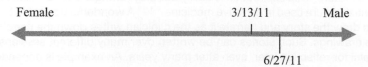

These figures can be collected and reviewed with the patient and family members over time in the ongoing assessment of gender identity.

Gender roadmaps—This is a term the author has used for a technique to help the individual visualize knowledge and goals and facilitate understanding of the variety of ways and how and when to reach these goals. Gender roadmaps are drawn by individuals in or between sessions to chart how they are proceeding and/or wish to proceed from their current gender to their desired gender. The roadmaps take into account the many different ways to get from one point to the other; the possible obstacles or catalysts that exist and may be encountered such as opposition from others, funding, and insurance and life events and situations such as school, vacations, and work. Impediments or facilitators can be listed alongside the roads connecting points along the way. These descriptors are used similarly to the linking phrases in concept maps[42] to give relationships to the conceptualized goals or destinations, allowing for adaptation to changing circumstances and shifting desires and identity as knowledge, particularly about practical aspects of transitioning, increases. A very simple example follows, with the linking words written horizontally.

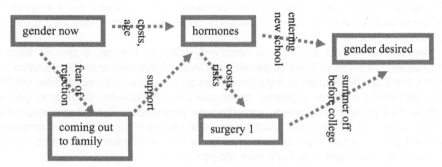

The author has found the use of individual gender roadmaps to be extraordinarily helpful in working with patients and their families. The roadmaps can be basic pencil-and-paper drawings or done on electronic media; some have used concept map Web sites for generating more formal roadmaps, although this is not necessary and is frequently unwieldy. These roadmaps are an example of generative learning and can be modified and redrawn at any time according to changes in the person's circumstances or identity. They can be relatively simple or very complex and creative, generating increased communication and understanding. Upon reaching or achieving each destination or goal, the roadmap can be redrawn to incorporate how that goal may alter the ongoing trajectory of transitioning.

The idea of a roadmap to help with decision-making for gender transitioning has also been used, although in an outline format, by Andrea James on the Web site www.tsroadmap.com.

For younger gender variant children in the stages of preoperational or concrete operations, most of whom will not be transgender in adolescence or adulthood, a concept similar to gender roadmaps can help them explore their fantasies and goals about their future. This exploration is easily done by having the child make up stories, an essential feature used in narrative medicine.[43,44] A wonderful way to do this is have the child draw the story and narrate it as the clinician writes down the narrative along with the drawings. Such stories can be written over many different sessions and are very useful for reflection later, even after many years. An example is appended at the end of this article (Appendix 1).

LGBT versus *T* versus *LG*—When writing about lesbian, gay, bisexual, and transgender issues, many have become comfortable using the abbreviation *LGBT*. However, the term is often used in a knee-jerk response even when not all parts of the abbreviation apply. For example, in 2011, one often heard the media and others use LGBT when referring to marriage equality debates or in the "don't ask, don't tell" (DADT) policy changes of the US military, even though these issues or debates most often did not encompass transgender (and/or bisexual) people. The elimination of

DADT in the summer of 2011 did not clarify how or if transgender or transsexual people can be in the military. Some people erroneously assume that transgender people are included in policy issues affecting only lesbian and gay people or that transgender people's needs are met by lesbian and gay organizations, whereas not all do. Although many services for transgender people originated in and/or are still part of organizations originally focused on lesbian and gay people, some transgender people believe that services in such LG organizations are not appropriate for them or do not meet their needs, especially if the name of the organization is not inclusive of transgender people. This incongruity is even more the case for transgender people who are attracted to people of another sex other than their own gender identity, because they do not, of course, consider themselves to be lesbian or gay.

To be even more inclusive, variations of the abbreviations *LGBTQ* or *LGBTQI* have been used to include questioning (Q) and intersex (I) people. The inclusion of "questioning" can be helpful for teenagers who are not yet certain of their sexual orientation or gender identity and for their parents who are not sure if LGBT services are appropriate for their children.

Sex reassignment, gender reassignment—These terms are also often used interchangeably, like *sex* and *gender* sometimes are, for procedures and changes one makes to become the other sex or gender; however, some use *gender reassignment* for changes one makes in clothing, hair, jewelry, voice, mannerisms, and so on and *sex reassignment* for biological changes using puberty suspension, exogenous hormones, and surgical procedures. Some prefer the terms *gender (*or *sex) correction* or *corrective* for steps or procedures planned/taken, as in correction of the body to fit the primacy of the identity. The process of reassignment or correction is generally referred to as transitioning.

Transvestite, cross-dressers, drag queen, drag king—In psychiatry, *transvestite* is shorthand for the diagnosis of transvestic disorder or transvestic fetishism with recurrent and intense sexual arousal from cross-dressing that gives distress and/or impairs functioning. Whereas this condition most commonly arises in adolescence, it is not a topic of this issue of the *Clinics*.

In common parlance, *transvestite* refers to anyone dressing and behaving as the other sex, which can be for pleasure but not necessarily (often not) erotic pleasure, for occupational reasons, or for shock or comedic value (and sometimes on only few occasions). Cross-dressers often dress as the other sex when opportunities arise to do so and usually engage in their regular activities of daily living while cross-dressed. *Drag queen* refers to a male performer dressed as female; *drag king* to a female performer dressed as male. Some contemporary well-known people who have engaged in transvestism and/or are drag entertainers include Rudolph Giuliani, Dennis Rodman, Eddie Murphy, RuPaul Andre Charles, Lypsinka (John Epperson), Murray Hill (Betsey Gallagher), Dame Edna Everage (Barry Humphries), Divine (Harris Glenn Milstead), Joey Arias, Eddie Izzard, Harvey Fierstein, John Travolta, and Alice Cooper. Entertainers who have crossed gender boundaries in their acts can be considered to have been engaged in transvestism, including David Bowie, members of the band Kiss, Annie Lennox, Boy George, and Prince, among many others.

Some cross-dressers or drag queens/kings may also identify as transgender and may procure varying degrees of biological transition; one example is the performer Justin Vivian Bond, who formerly performed in drag as Kiki (of Kiki and Herb), and currently uses the pronoun V and goes by the middle name Vivian and honorific Mx.

Sexual identity—This term is often used by someone who is struggling to understand another's sexual orientation or gender identity. When someone refers a patient to the author for sexual identity problems, it is not known if the patient is having trouble with his/her sexual orientation or gender identity, and the author gathers that the referring clinician did not have the time or the expertise to parse this further. Some experts in the field consider sexual identity to be the gestalt of a person's sexual orientation, sexual behavior, gender identity, plus gender role.

Intersex, disorders of sexual development—Intersex conditions, or commonly now referred to as disorders of sexual development (DSD), were previously known as *hermaphroditism* or *pseudohermaphroditism*, archaic and confusing terms. People with DSD have congenitally abnormal, intermediate, and/or unformed physical features of being male or female. The most commonly found DSD is congenital adrenal hyperplasia; others are androgen insensitivity syndrome, 5-α-reductase-2 deficiency, 17-β-hydroxysteroid dehydrogenase III deficiency, cloacal or bladder exstrophy, mosaicism, and chimerism.

A BRIEF HISTORY OF GENDER VARIANCE IN YOUTH

Although a historical survey of gender variance and transgenderism is beyond the scope of this *Clinics* issue, these uncommon facets of humankind have been present and reported since earliest times. Various societies have managed these facets in widely different ways, from open acceptance and accommodation with important social roles for gender variant and transgender people to hostility and persecution. A number of sources give extensive histories in this regard and should be investigated for a more complete understanding of the human condition. Gil Herdt's encyclopedic tome, *Third Sex, Third Gender: Beyond Sexual Dimorphism in Culture and History*,[45] has erudite discussions of eunuchs, the mahu and fa'afafine of Polynesia, the Native American berdache, and the hijra of India. Leslie Feinberg's seminal *Transgender Warriors: Making History from Joan of Arc to Dennis Rodman*,[46] is an essential reference. Susan Stryker's *Transgender History*[47] is an accessible review of American transgender history from the mid-20th century on and is an excellent book for teens and young adults. Joanne Meyerowitz's *How Sex Changed: A History of Transsexuality in the United States*[48] is also an important reference.

The history of the treatment of gender variance in youth has been controversial, with both the therapeutic techniques and the goals of treatment coming into question. Clinicians have been criticized for using such behavioral strategies as punishment, coercion, and religious persuasion with children. Criticism has also been merited for some clinicians who have promised or endorsed goals of altering a child's later sexual orientation (ie, preventing homosexuality) or gender identity (ie, preventing transgenderism). Discussions of these issues can be found in several articles in this *Clinics* issue as well as elsewhere in the literature.[37–39]

Despite, or because of the clinical and cultural complexities and the controversies and challenges of working with gender variant children and transgender adolescents, there is a shortage of mental health professionals with training or experience in these issues, and a disparity of care exists.[49] Currently, there are fewer than a dozen child and adolescent psychiatrists in North America who can be regarded having a degree of expertise in this area; many are contributors to this *Clinics* issue. There are not a great many more psychologists, social workers, or nurses in this regard either. Early pioneers and recent and newer experts in working with gender variant and transgender youth in the United States include John Money, PhD (deceased); Richard Green, MD, JD; Heino Meyer-Bahlburg, Dr rer nat (a contributor to this issue); Anke Ehrhardt, PhD; Susan Coates, PhD; Richard Stoller, MD (deceased); Bernard Zuger, MD; Dennis Anderson, MD (deceased); William Womack, MD; William Stone, MD (deceased); Sarah Herbert, MD, MSW (a contributor to this issue); Catherine Tuerk, MA, RN (a contributor to this issue); Edgardo Menvielle, MD (a contributor to this issue); William

Reiner, MD (a contributor to this issue); Stewart Adelson MD (a contributor to this issue); Scott Leibowitz, MD (a contributor to this issue); Joel Stoddard, MD, MAS (a contributor to this issue); and this author, as well as the endocrinologists Wylie Hembree, MD, and Norman Spack, MD (both contributors to this issue). In Toronto, these mental health experts include Susan Bradley, MD; Kenneth Zucker, PhD (a contributor to this issue); and Solomon Shapiro, MD. In the Netherlands, these include Peggy Cohen-Kettenis, PhD, and Annelou de Vries, MD, PhD (both contributors to this issue). In England, this includes Domenic Di Ceglie, MD, at the Tavistock Clinic. The writings of these experts who are not contributors to this issue can be easily searched. These named individuals have added to the understanding and care of gender variant and transgender youth, and most have worked within their own and in other professional organizations to advance policies and procedures to improve such patient care.

SELECTED PROFESSIONAL ORGANIZATIONS' HISTORIES AND POLICIES ON LGBT MATTERS

This section highlights the history of how LGBT matters have been addressed by several of the major professional psychiatric organizations in the United States as well as several other pertinent national and international ones. Most of these organizations have been on the forefront of advocating for the care and well-being of LGBT people and continue to be crucial in supporting and educating mental health professionals to improve such care. Heath care needs regarding gender identity issues for gender variant, transgender, transsexual, and intersex people have followed subsequent to (albeit more slowly than) the seminal advances made for lesbian and gay people since the gay rights movement burgeoned in North America, proceeding from the Stonewall riots in New York City in 1969 and other similar civil rights protests around the country in the 1960s to 1980s.

American Psychiatric Association

The American Psychiatric Association (APA) since 1973 has had position statements that oppose discrimination on the basis of sexual orientation, and "opposes any psychiatric treatment, such as reparative or conversion therapy which is based upon the assumption that homosexuality per se is a mental disorder or based upon the a priori assumption that the patient should change his/her sexual homosexual orientation."[50] This opposition could presumably be applied to gender variant children who are being treated with the goal of the prevention of homosexuality. In 1973, the APA removed homosexuality as a mental disorder from the third edition of the Diagnostic Manual of Mental Disorders.[30] Also see the following Reports and Initiatives section for information on current APA initiatives. Several authors in this issue are APA members.

Association of Gay and Lesbian Psychiatrists

In the 1960s, gay and lesbian members of the APA met informally at the annual APA meetings. The Caucus of Gay, Lesbian, and Bisexual Members of the American Psychiatric Association (formerly the Caucus of Homosexual-Identified Psychiatrists) was established in the mid 1970s; in 1985, the caucus changed its name to the Association of Gay and Lesbian Psychiatrists (AGLP) as an affiliated but separate organization to the APA, and as such it issues positions independent of the APA. In 1986, AGLP was instrumental in the removal of the prejudicial diagnosis of ego-dystonic homosexuality from the revised DSM. AGLP represents hundreds of psychiatrists, other health care professionals or concerned individuals, and trainees; the organization educates and advocates on lesbian, gay, bisexual, and transgender mental health issues. The primary annual AGLP meeting is during the APA annual meeting; many topics promoting transgender health have been covered. Since its founding, AGLP has sponsored many presentations on LGBT care for the APA's scientific proceedings. Several authors in this issue are AGLP members.

American Academy of Child and Adolescent Psychiatry

The American Academy of Child and Adolescent Psychiatry (AACAP), representing approximately 7000 child and adolescent psychiatrists and trainees in the United States, approved their policy statement on sexual orientation and civil rights in 1992, opposing discrimination based on sexual orientation, and another on gay and lesbian parenting in 1999. These were updated and approved in 2009 to be more encompassing and inclusive of gender variant children and adolescents and transgender parents.[51,52] The revised 2009 policy statements, on sexual orientation, gender identity, and civil rights and on gay, lesbian, bisexual, or transgender parents include the following language: AACAP "*rejects* all public and private discrimination based on sexual orientation or gender identity of persons of any age .... AACAP affirms the right of all people to their orientation and identity without interference or coercive interventions attempting to change sexual orientation or gender identity ..."[51]; AACAP "opposes any discrimination based on sexual orientation or gender identity against individuals in regard to their rights as custodial, foster, or adoptive parents."[52] These policy statements are useful in advocacy efforts; they can be found at www.aacap.org. Also, see the following Reports and Initiatives section for information on current AACAP initiatives. Six authors in this issue are AACAP members: Drs Reiner, Pleak, Herbert, Menvielle, Stoddard, and Leibowitz.

Lesbian and Gay Child and Adolescent Psychiatric Association and Sexual Orientation and Gender Identity Issues Committee

In 1989 and 1990, several gay and lesbian child and adolescent psychiatrists founded the Lesbian and Gay Child and Adolescent Psychiatric Association (LAGCAPA) as an affiliated but separate group to AACAP. LAGCAPA quickly grew to become an international organization representing well over one hundred child and adolescent psychiatrists and trainees. The mission of LAGCAPA is multifold: to educate our profession about LGBT youth, to advocate for LGBT youth and eliminate discrimination, to support LGBT child and adolescent psychiatrists and trainees, to encourage research and foster education, and to promote the welfare of LGBT youth (see www.lagcapa.org). LAGCAPA meets during the annual AACAP meeting; members include both LGBT– and non-LGBT–identified professionals who support the LAGCAPA mission. Five authors in this issue are LAGCAPA members: Drs Pleak, Herbert, Menvielle, Stoddard, and Leibowitz; the first three have also served as LAGCAPA presidents.

Under the initiative and advocacy of LAGCAPA/AACAP members and on the invitation and encouragement of the AACAP Executive Council in the mid-1990s, the Homosexual Issues Committee was formed as an official component of AACAP; the committee's name was changed in 2003 to the Sexual Orientation and Gender Identity Issues Committee (SOGIIC). SOGIIC membership overlaps with LAGCAPA membership to a certain extent and also includes non-LGBT–identified AACAP members. SOGIIC works within the AACAP with its mission to serve in an educational and research advisory capacity to the AACAP membership concerning issues involving LGBT children and adolescents and their families, to serve in an advisory capacity to the AACAP concerning professional issues for LGBT child psychiatry residents and members, and to actively promote the development of the database and educational curricula concerning LGBT issues in child and adolescent psychiatry;

this involvement includes revising and updating AACAP policy statements. Five authors in this issue are SOGIIC members: Drs Pleak (SOGIIC Chair through October 2011), Herbert (SOGIIC Chair as of October 2011), Menvielle, Stoddard, and Leibowitz.

SOGIIC and LAGCAPA work together in developing scientific programs on LGBT issues for presentation at AACAP, APA, World Professional Association for Transgender Health (WPATH), and other international and local meetings; SOGIIC and LAGCAPA have worked together on the AACAP Practice Parameters on LGBT youth (see article by Adelson in this issue) and have sponsored several hundred symposia, workshops, clinical consultations, institutes, papers, posters, media theaters, grand rounds, and other presentations at such meetings since 1990; many of these have focused on gender variant children and transgender adolescents.

Gay and Lesbian Medical Association

The Gay and Lesbian Medical Association (GLMA) is the world's largest and oldest association of LGBT health care professionals. GLMA was founded in 1981 as the American Association of Physicians for Human Rights. GLMA's mission is to ensure equality in health care for lesbian, gay, bisexual, and transgender individuals and health care providers; the organization represents the interests of tens of thousands of LGBT health professionals of all kinds, as well as millions of LGBT patients. The Healthcare Equality Index (HEI) is a joint project of GLMA and the Human Rights Campaign Foundation.[53] The HEI provides a quality indicator for health care related to lesbian, gay, bisexual, and transgender people, beginning with the hospital industry. The survey focuses on specific hospital policies in several areas: patient nondiscrimination, hospital visitation, decision-making, cultural competency training for hospital staff, and hospital employment policies.

American Medical Association

The American Medical Association (AMA) has policies inclusive of the rights of transgender persons.[54] These AMA Policies include the following:

- Eliminating Health Disparities—Promoting Awareness and Education of LGBT Health Issues in Medical Education
- Removing Financial Barriers to Care for Transgender Patients
- Health Disparities Among Gay, Lesbian, Bisexual and Transgender Families
- Civil Rights Restoration
- Health Care Needs of the Homosexual Population
- Patient-Physician Relationship: Respect for Law and Human Rights
- Civil Rights and Professional Responsibility
- Potential Patients.

These AMA policies can be accessed at www.ama-assn.org.

Harry Benjamin International Gender Dysphoria Association/World Professional Association for Transgender Health

The first major international organization of professionals caring for transgender people was formed in 1979 as the Harry Benjamin International Gender Dysphoria Association (HBIGDA). The name gave tribute to Dr Harry Benjamin (1885–1986), a German-American endocrinologist and sexologist who was a pioneer in helping transsexual people. Benjamin treated many transsexual patients including Christine Jorgensen, and he wrote the influential 1966 book, *The Transsexual Phenomenon*.[55] In 2008, HBIGDA officially changed its name to the World Professional Association for

Transgender Health. WPATH members include professionals in fields such as endocrinology, psychiatry, surgery, psychology, law, social work, family studies, sociology, anthropology, speech and voice therapy, and sexology, as well as individuals who do not work in these professional disciplines; WPATH includes many transgender members.

WPATH developed and published its first treatment guidelines as the HBIGDA Standards of Care for Gender Identity Disorders (SoC) in 1979; this is the organization's professional consensus about the psychiatric, psychological, medical, and surgical management of gender identity disorders. SoC updates were published in 1980, 1981, 1990, and 1998, with the current sixth version published in 2001.[56] A seventh version of SoC is in development and is planned to be available in 2011 or 2012 under the organization's WPATH name. WPATH holds biennial symposia; the 21st Biennial Symposium in Oslo, Norway, in June 2009, titled Childhood-Adulthood: Culture and Brain, was focused on children and adolescents as well as on feedback about the proposed gender identity disorder diagnosis revision in DSM-5; seven authors in this issue are WPATH members and attended and presented at the Oslo meeting: Drs Meyer-Bahlburg, Zucker, Cohen-Kettenis, Herbert, Menvielle, Steensma, and Pleak; Drs de Vries is also a member. WPATH's 22nd Biennial Symposium, Transgender Beyond Disorder: Identity, Community, and Health, is in September 2011 in Atlanta, Georgia, in conjunction with the Southern Comfort Conference, the largest transgender community conference in the United States, and the Gay and Lesbian Medical Association's Annual Conference. Conference proceedings for WPATH can be found at www.wpath.org.

National Association for Research and Therapy of Homosexuality

The National Association for Research and Therapy of Homosexuality (NARTH) was founded in 1992 as the National Association for Research and Treatment of Homosexuality by three psychoanalysts: the late psychiatrist Charles Socarides, psychiatrist Benjamin Kaufman, and psychologist Joseph Nicolosi, "in response to the growing threat of scientific censorship." NARTH states that it "offers hope to those who struggle with unwanted homosexuality"; it believes that homosexuality is not normal, natural, or healthy, disagreeing with the APA's removal of homosexuality from the DSM in 1973.[31] NARTH earlier openly advocated for the treatment of "pre-homosexual" children (equivalent as "gender-disturbed" children to NARTH) to prevent them from becoming homosexual, despite no evidence that any treatment alters later sexual orientation. The organization states that in current times, "Gender-disturbed children are no longer helped to become more comfortable with their own biological sex, or with the same-sex peers they have been avoiding"[57]. NARTH advocates for so-called reparative therapy of homosexual people in order to change "unwanted" sexual orientation and behavior. This reparative therapy has been judged by most experts to lack evidence for effectiveness and to be potentially harmful; as such, it has been repudiated by the APA, the American Psychological Association, the AACAP, the American Psychoanalytic Association, and many other professional organizations.

Another longtime and leading member of NARTH has been the psychologist George Rekers, who was active in the early studies of the behavioral treatment of gender-referred boys since the 1970s, with the goal of preventing homosexuality and transsexualism.[58,59] Rekers evoked controversy in the 1980s and 1990s when he openly called homosexuality "a sin," "a disorder," "degenerative," and "proscribed by the Ten Commandments" and authored several religious and other press books concerned with the prevention of homosexuality.[60–62] Rekers, regarded as a nationally prominent antigay activist, again courted controversy in May 2010 when newspapers reported his having hired a 20-year-old male prostitute to go with him on vacation for two weeks.[63] After this scandal he was no longer listed as listed as a NARTH advisor and officer, and resigned from its board.

Intersex Society of North America/Accord Alliance

As e-mail and the Internet increased the ease and rapidity of contact of people with relatively uncommon conditions, organizations to meet their needs organized or grew swiftly; e-mail and Internet communities of intersex people became accessible in the 1990s. The Intersex Society of North America (ISNA) was founded in 1993 to advocate for intersex patients and their families (see www.isna.org). ISNA held an unofficial gathering during the 1997 meeting of the APA in San Diego; about 30 psychiatrists attended (including the author) to hear ISNA founder Cheryl Chase's plea for improved care for intersex children, such as postponing nonessential surgical procedures involving sex and reassignment of natal sex until the child grows to an age to make his/her own decisions about these matters, ending unwanted (and difficult to reverse) genital surgeries. Although initially seen as a radical and fringe group whose newsletter was provocatively called *Hermaphrodites with Attitude*, ISNA became respected, and many of its recommendations are now commonplace in the surgical and psychiatric management of intersex children. ISNA closed down in 2008 after convening a national group of health care and advocacy professionals to establish a nonprofit organization known as the Accord Alliance, with its mission to improve DSD-related health care and outcomes (see www.accordalliance.org). The Accord Alliance is a helpful resource for intersex people and their families.

RECENT REPORTS AND INITIATIVES REGARDING GENDER IDENTITY

The first national, representative survey of transgender people was published in 2011. This report, *Injustice at Every Turn: A Report of the National Transgender Discrimination Survey*,[64] documents pervasive discrimination against transgender people. Key survey findings were that suicide attempts were reported by 41% of the 6450 respondents; 78% reported harassment and 35% reported physical assault while in school (K–12), and 15% left school because of harassment. Antitransgender bias coupled with persistent racism was most devastating. Not surprisingly then, respondents had double the general population's rate of unemployment, with poverty four times the national average; 47% had an adverse job outcome (fired, not hired, denied promotion) due to gender identity/expression; 50% were harassed on the job; and 71% attempted to avoid discrimination by hiding their gender or transition. Healthier findings that inform possible prevention were that 78% who had transitioned to the other sex felt more comfortable and had improved job performance; 76% had been able to receive hormone therapy; and many who had to leave school later returned to school, with high numbers (22%) of 25- to 44-year-olds in school. The report implicates nearly "every system and institution in the United States . . . [for] failing in its obligation to serve transgender and gender non-conforming people instead of subjecting them to mistreatment ranging from common-place disrespect to outright violence, abuse and the denial of human dignity," the consequences of which are "ranging from unemployment and homelessness to illness and death." The report is a "call to action for all of us" to "take up the call for human rights for transgender and gender non-conforming people, and confront this pattern of abuse and injustice."[64] The survey included people from all 50 states, the District of Columbia, Puerto Rico, Guam, and the US Virgin Islands.

The medical profession is being asked to become more knowledgeable about LGBT people. The highly influential Institute of Medicine (IoM) issued a groundbreaking report in March 2011 titled, *The Heath of Lesbian, Gay, Bisexual, and Transgender*

People: Building a Foundation for Better Understanding.[65] This report recognized the dearth of data on LGBT people and the past and current limitations on funding such research. The report called for an increase in research on LGBT populations with increased participation of sexual and gender minorities in research, with a goal to "not only benefit LGBT individuals, but also add to the repository of health information we have that pertains to all people."[65] The IoM works to provide unbiased and authoritative advice to decision makers and the public; the IoM reports are used to direct change in medical education, policies, and practice.

The *Healthcare Equality Index 2011: Creating a National Standard for Equal Treatment of Lesbian, Gay, Bisexual and Transgender Patients and Their Families*,[53] conducted and published by the Human Rights Campaign Foundation and endorsed by the GLMA, found that over 40% of surveyed health care organizations do not yet protect transgender patients from discrimination, nearly half do not train all their personnel on LGBT cultural competency, and an even smaller number require this training.[65] This report relied on self-report from 375 respondents from 29 states and the District of Columbia. Therefore, the majority of United States health care organizations did not respond, and presumably the national rates of protection and training on the basis on gender identity and expression are much lower.

The Joint Commission (JC), the major organization that accredits and certifies health care organizations and programs in the United States, thusly has a paramount influence on health care policies and practice. The JC, in its 2010 publication, *Advancing Effective Communication, Cultural Competence, and Patient- and Family-Centered Care: A Roadmap for Hospitals*, recognizes the impact of—and disparities in—health care due to gender identity issues.[66] The JC recommends that hospitals should develop new or modify existing policies and procedures to protect patients from discrimination based on their sexual orientation and gender identity or expression and that hospitals should define family to explicitly include any individual that plays a significant role in the patient's life such as spouse, domestic partner, significant other (of different sex or same-sex), or other individual not legally related to the patient. The JC also recommends that hospitals protect staff from discrimination based on sexual orientation or gender identity or expression. In general, the JC will soon require that hospitals prohibit discrimination based on sexual orientation and gender identity or expression. Since few United States health care organizations and programs, including most medical schools, prohibit discrimination based on gender identity and expression,[65] this JC requirement will stimulate these organizations to develop and implement such policies and to instruct staff and trainees in these issues. Institutions will likely seek out mental health professionals to assist in this effort to comply with these new regulations.

The University of California, San Francisco (UCSF) Center for LGBT Health and Equity is currently the only LGBT office in a health setting in the United States. This Center held the first ever National Summit on LGBT Issues in Medical Education in September 2010, attended by over 80 health care educators (including the author) and administrators from across the United States and was chaired by Shane Snowdon, the center's director and a contributor to this issue. The aim of the summit was to foster the development of other LGBT centers (or at least augment resources) across the country in order to improve support to and address the concerns and needs of LGBT trainees, faculty, staff, and patients in medical schools and health care facilities and to provide training to and promote the care of LGBT patients by non-LGBT trainees, faculty, and staff. For further information and for the UCSF Center's excellent curriculum resources, see http://lgbt.ucsf.edu.

Appendix 1

A Child's Storybook (Figs. 1–8)

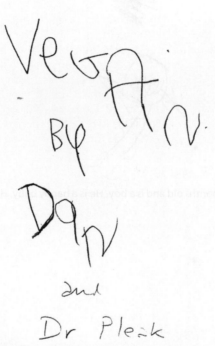

Fig. 1. Title: *Vegan,* by Dan and Dr Pleak. A Narrative Story about Gender Identity by a 5-Year-Old Natal Male Over 7 Sessions. [Note: "Dan" drew this story with the author writing down Dan's narrative after he had been in therapy with the author for about a year.]

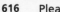

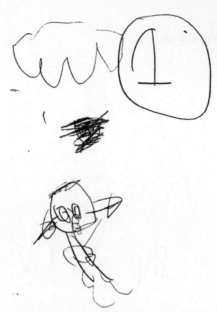

Fig. 2. Baby Vegan is 3 months old and is a boy. He is a happy baby. He draws pictures and saw it raining.

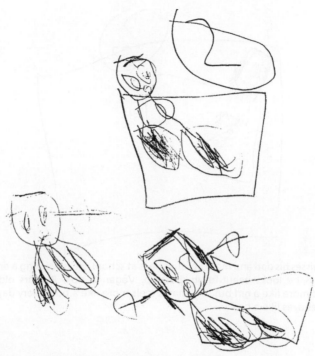

Fig. 3. Vegan is 3 years old and is wearing big socks, a diaper, and a big girl's dress. His mother is happy the baby's out and the father wished he could live with Vegan because he is moving out and he is sad. Vegan is a boy but sometimes feels he is a girl. [Note: Father and mother were becoming estranged at this time of "Dan's" therapy.]

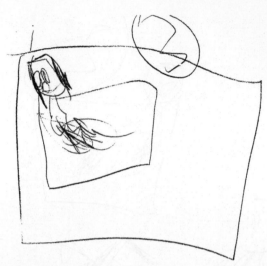

Fig. 4. Vegan misses his dad and mom because he is at school. He is wearing a dress in school. The teacher says he looks beautiful in dress-up. Vegan is now 8 years old. Vegan still sometimes feels more like a girl but sometimes feels more like a boy. Every day he takes his dress off and behaves like a boy.

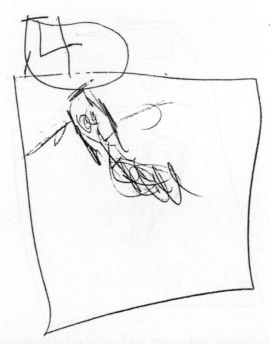

Fig. 5. Vegan is a smart teenager in high school, but he's off today and is home on vacation. He is wearing pants and a shirt. Vegan doesn't like to be a girl anymore. He doesn't wear girls' dresses—he would be teased in high school if he did. His best friends are Danielle and Dans.

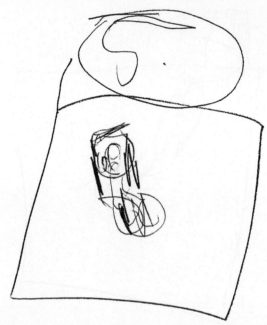

Fig. 6. Vegan is still a teenager and is home sick from school. If he was well, he would color. He is not dating.

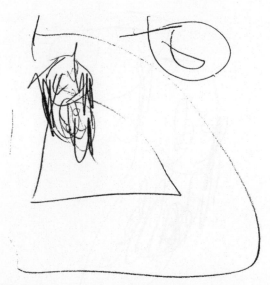

Fig. 7. Vegan is a still a teenager. He is in school and about to go home. He wondered to his mom, "could I read the Jungle Book?", and tells her, "I love you so much." He sees his father for the first time in a very long time and says "I wondered where you were so long." [Note: the father was in the process of moving out of the home, and the mother was terminally ill and would die a year after this story was written.]

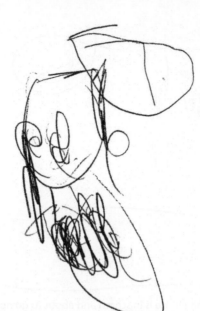

Fig. 8. Vegan is grown-up—he is an adult man. He is working as an ice-skater helper. He lives with Dr Mellon, a man. He doesn't yet have kids, but might have a baby out of his belly (he's faking!). His mommy and daddy finally visited him in his new house—he forgot to tell them where he moved! [Note: "Dan" is now 21 years old and still seen by the author on occasion for medication of his mild psychiatric disorder; he is studying abroad in college and identifies as a bisexual male; he reports no desire to be female since he was 5 or 6 years old. He and the author have looked at this story every several years and are both surprised at how prescient young "Dan" was back then.]

REFERENCES

1. Bono C. Transition: the story of how I became a man. New York: Dutton Adult; 2011.
2. Drath E. Renée. Bristol (CT): ESPN; 2011.
3. Turnbull L. Kids challenge gender identity earlier—and get support. Seattle Times; July 30, 2011.
4. Hoffman J. Boys will be boys? Not in these families. New York Times; June 10, 2011.
5. Zolotow C, Pene Du Bois W. William's doll. New York: Harper & Row; 1985.
6. Sachar L, Sullivan B. Is he a girl? New York: Random House Books for Young Readers; 1993.
7. Jennings K, Shapiro P. Always my child: a parent's guide to understanding your gay, lesbian, bisexual, transgender, or questioning son or daughter. Los Angeles: Fireside Press; 2002.
8. Xavier J, Boenke M, Lev AI. Trans forming families: real stories about transgendered loved ones. 2nd edition. New Castle (DE): Oak Knoll Press; 2003.
9. Peters JA. Luna. New York: Little, Brown Books for Young Readers; 2006.
10. Winfield C. Gender identity: the ultimate teen guide (it happened to me). Lanham (MD): Scarecrow Press; 2006.
11. Evelyn J. Mom, I need to be a girl. North Charleston (SC): Booksurge Publishing; 2007.
12. Pascoe CJ. Dude, you're a fag: masculinity and sexuality in high school. Berkeley (CA): University of California Press; 2007.

13. Beam C. Transparent: love, family, and living the T with transgender teens. New York; Houghton Mifflin Harcourt; 2008.
14. Brill SA, Pepper R. The transgender child: a handbook for families and professionals. Berkeley (CA): Cleis Press, 2008.
15. Ewert M, Ray R. 10,000 dresses. New York: Seven Stories Press; 2008.
16. Stockton KB. The queer child, or growing sideways in the twentieth century. Durham (NC): Duke University Press Books; 2009.
17. Carr J, Rumback B. Be who you are. Bloomington (IN): AuthorHouse; 2010.
18. Kilodavis C, DeSimone S. My princess boy. New York: Aladdin; 2010.
19. McIntosh K, Walker I. Youth with gender issues: seeking an identity (helping youth with mental, physical, and social challenges). Broomall (PA): Mason Crest Publishers; 2010.
20. Nagle J. Teens: being gay, lesbian, bisexual, or transgender: GLBT teens and society. New York: Rosen Publishing; 2010.
21. Orr TB. Teens: being gay, lesbian, bisexual, or transgender: home and family relationships. New York: Rosen Publishing; 2010.
22. Payment S. Teens: being gay, lesbian, bisexual, or transgender: friendship, dating, and relationships. New York: Rosen Publishing; 2010.
23. Worth R. Teens: Being gay, lesbian, bisexual, or transgender: life at school and the community. New York: Rosen Publishing; 2010.
24. Seba JA. Feeling wrong in your own body: understanding what it means to be transgender (Gallup's guide to modern gay, lesbian and transgender lifestyle). Broomall (PA): Mason Crest Publishers; 2010.
25. Beam C. I am J. New York: Little, Brown Books for Young Readers; 2011.
26. Ehrensaft D. Gender born, gender made: raising healthy gender-nonconforming children. New York: The Experiment; 2011.
27. Krieger I. Helping your transgender teen: a guide for parents. New Haven (CT): Genderwise Press; 2011.
28. Huegel K. GLBTQ: The survival guide for gay, lesbian, bisexual, transgender, and questioning teens. Minneapolis (MN): Free Spirit Publishing; 2011.
29. Rothblatt P. All I want to be is me. On-Demand Publishing: CreateSpace; 2011.
30. Savage D, Miller T. It gets better: coming out, overcoming bullying, and creating a life worth living. New York: Dutton Adult; 2011.
31. Bayer R. Homosexuality and American psychiatry. Princeton (NJ): Princeton University Press; 1987.
32. American Psychiatric Association. DSM-5; the future of psychiatric diagnosis. DSM-5 development Web site. http://www.dsm5.org. Accessed August 14, 2011,
33. American Psychiatric Association. Diagnostic and statistical manual of mental disorders. 3rd edition. Washington, DC: American Psychiatric Association; 1981.
34. American Psychiatric Association. Diagnostic and statistical manual of mental disorders. 3rd edition revised. Washington, DC: American Psychiatric Association; 1987.
35. American Psychiatric Association. Diagnostic and statistical manual of mental disorders. 4th edition, text revision. Washington, DC: American Psychiatric Association; 2000.
36. World Health Organization. International statistical classification of diseases and related health problems. 10th revision, version for 2007. http://apps.who.int/classifications/apps/icd/icd10online. Accessed August 14, 2011.
37. Pleak RR. Ethical issues in the treatment of gender atypical children and adolescents. In: Rottnek M, editor. Sissies and tomboys: gender nonconformity and homosexual childhood. New York: New York University Press; 1999. p. 34–51.
38. Pleak RR. Formation of transgender identities in adolescence. Journal of Gay and Lesbian Mental Health 2009;13:282–291.

39. Pleak RR. Treating gender variant children and adolescents. Presented at World Professional Association for Transgender Health Biennial Symposium. Oslo, Norway. June, 2009.

40. Steiner BW, editor. Gender dysphoria: development, research, management. New York: Plenum Press; 1985.

41. Diamond LA. Sexual Fluidity: Understanding Women's Love and Desire. Cambridge: Harvard University Press, 2008.

42. Fornari A. Clarifying with concept maps. Faculty education workshop at Hofstra North Shore-LIJ School of Medicine, Hempstead (NY), 2011.

43. Peterkin A. Why we write (and how we can do it better). CMAJ 2010;182(15): 1650–2.

44. Charon R. Narrative medicine: a model for empathy, reflection, profession, and trust. JAMA 2001;286(15):1897–1902.

45. Herdt G, editor. Third sex, third gender: beyond sexual dimorphism in culture and history. New York: Zone Books; 1994.

46. Feinberg L. Transgender warriors: making history from Joan of Arc to Dennis Rodman. Boston (MA): Beacon Press; 1997.

47. Stryker S. Transgender history. Berkeley (CA): Seal Press; 2008.

48. Meyerowitz J. How sex changed: a history of transsexuality in the United States. Cambridge (MA): Harvard University Press; 2004.

49. Pleak RR. Transgender persons. In: Pedro Ruiz P, Primm A, editors. Disparities in psychiatric care: clinical and cross-cultural perspectives. Philadelphia: Lippincott Williams & Wilkins; 2010.

50. American Psychiatric Association. Therapies focused on attempts to change sexual orientation (reparative or conversion therapies). Position statement. American Psychiatric Association Web site. http://www.psych.org/Departments/EDU/Library/APAOfficial DocumentsandRelated/PositionStatements/200001.aspx. Accessed August 14, 2011. Published 2011.

51. American Academy of Child and Adolescent Psychiatry. Sexual orientation, gender identity, and civil rights. http://www.aacap.org/cs/root/policy_statements/sexual_ orientation_gender_identity_and_civil_rights.

52. American Academy of Child and Adolescent Psychiatry. Gay, lesbian, bisexual, or transgender parents policy statement. Available at: http://www.aacap.org/cs/root/ policy_statements/gay_lesbian_transgender_and_bisexual_parents_policy_statement. Accessed August 14, 2011.

53. Delpercio A. Healthcare Equality Index 2011: creating a national standard for equal treatment of lesbian, gay, bisexual and transgender patients and their families. Washington, DC; Human Rights Campaign Foundation; 2011.

54. GLBT Advisory Committee. AMA policy regarding sexual orientation. American Medical Association Web site. Available at:http://www.ama-assn.org/ama/pub/about-ama/our-people/member-groups-sections/glbt-advisory-committee/ama-policy-regarding-sexual-orientation.page. Accessed August 14, 2011.

55. Benjamin H. The transsexual phenomenon. New York: The Julian Press; 1966.

56. Meyer M, Bockting W, Cohen-Kettenis PT, et al. Harry Benjamin International Gender Dysphoria Association's Standards of Care for Gender Identity Disorder. 6th version. International Journal of Transgenderism 2001; 5(1). Available at: http//www.wpath.org/ publications standards.cfm. Accessed August 14, 2011.

57. National Association for Research and Therapy of Homosexuality. Our purpose: defending true diversity. NARTH Web site. http://www.narth.com/menus/statement.html. Accessed August 14, 2011.

58. Rekers GA, Lovaas OI. Behavioral treatment of deviant sex-role behaviors in a male child. J Appl Behav Anal 1974;7(2):173–90.
59. Rekers GA. The purpose of treatment for gender disturbed boys. Personnel and Guidance Journal 1980;58:4550–2.
60. Rekers GA. Growing up straight: what families should know about homosexuality. Chicago: Moody Press; 1982.
61. Rekers GA. Shaping your child's sexual identity. Grand Rapids (MI): Baker Book House; 1982.
62. Rekers GA. Handbook of child and adolescent sexual problems. New York: Lexington Books; 1995.
63. Bullock P, Bullock P. Christian right leader George Rekers takes vacation with "rent boy." Miami New Times. May 6, 2010.
64. Grant JM, Mottet LA, Tanis J, et al. Injustice at every turn: a report of the National Transgender Discrimination Survey. Washington, DC: National Center for Transgender Equality and National Gay and Lesbian Task Force; 2011.
65. Institute of Medicine. The health of lesbian, gay, bisexual, and transgender people: building a foundation for better understanding. Washington, DC: The National Academies Press; 2011.
66. The Joint Commission: Advancing Effective Communication, Cultural Competence, and Patient- and Family-Centered Care: A roadmap for hospitals. Oakbrook Terrace (IL): The Joint Commission; 2010.

Thoughts on the Nature of Identity: Disorders of Sex Development and Gender Identity

William G. Reiner, MD[a,b,*], D. Townsend Reiner, MA[c]

KEYWORDS

- Gender identity • Disorders of sex development
- Developmental psychopathology • Gender dysphoria

The unfolding of the sense of identity is central to child development. Gender identity is woven pervasively throughout identity. To understand gender identity, we must understand aspects of child development and, similarly, aspects of sex development (as opposed to pubertal sexual development). This understanding is especially important when applied to children born with disorders of sex development (DSD, also known as intersex conditions). Children with DSD are typically identified at birth as having ambiguous genitalia; they demonstrate at birth marked fetal developmental genital anomalies. These genital anomalies inject a pronounced clinical complexity: assigning the neonate an appropriate sex of rearing.[1] Long-term outcome data for most children with DSD have been sparse. What might we expect if we were to review outcomes today? In this article we present clinical experience regarding outcomes of children with DSD whose neonatal assignment of sex-of-rearing used the traditional clinical criteria for decision-making.[1]

CHILD DEVELOPMENT IN DSD

Disorders of sex development is the deliberate term for a range of disorders of sexual differentiation, sex chromosomal anomalies, and embryonic-fetal anatomical anomalies of genital or reproductive organs.[1] As a field of research, this designation

The authors have nothing to disclose.

[a] Section of Pediatric Urology, Department of Urology, Division of Child and Adolescent Psychiatry (Adjunct), University of Oklahoma Health Sciences Center 920 Stanton L. Young Boulevard, WP 3150, Oklahoma City, OK 73104, USA
[b] Section of Pediatric Urology, Department of Psychiatry, Division of Child and Adolescent Psychiatry (Adjunct), University of Oklahoma Health Sciences Center, 920 Stanton L. Young Boulevard, WP 3150, Oklahoma City, OK 73104, USA
[c] 21 Brookline St #407, Cambridge MA 02139, USA
* Corresponding author.
E-mail address: william-reiner@ouhsc.edu

Child Adolesc Psychiatric Clin N Am 20 (2011) 627–638
doi:10.1016/j.chc.2011.07.007
1056-4993/11/$ – see front matter © 2011 Elsevier Inc. All rights reserved.

represents a 2005 consensus view of a committee of internationally recognized experts in intersex and related areas (the senior author, W.G.R., was a committee member). It is certainly a welcome addition to a field that has been sorely lacking in expertise. Indeed, definitional inconsistency at the social and clinical levels, insufficient nosology, and a lack of precision in assessments and interventions from clinic to clinic are among the grosser inadequacies that the consensus committee sought to address through the establishment of its report as a baseline for more coherent research and consistent clinical applications.

Both research and clinical approaches are important. Indeed, the clinical conundrum in the neonate with a DSD, this unknown of the child's future identity or ultimate recognized gender, can provide unusual insights into the development of the sexual self. This insight might have clinical and research implications for gender identity development as well as sexual orientation, even if within the confines of the atypical conditions. This area of study is particularly relevant, as the *Diagnostic and Statistical Manual of Mental Disorders, fifth edition*[2] (DSM-5) Sexual and Gender Identity Disorders Work Group of the American Psychiatric Association is in the process of actively revising and testing new formulations for psychiatric diagnoses: gender identity disorder (GID) and its relationship to DSD are among those topics being considered for revision in the new manual. Questions concerning gender dysphoria in children with DSD and in children with GID have led some to wonder how these two disorders might be related, at least in terms of gender dysphoria. (In this discussion the term *gender dysphoria* is a term that will be used to describe either DSD or GID.) An additional question has been raised within the DSM-5 Work Group and by some clinicians, patient support groups, and others as to whether GID is a de facto psychopathology at all.[3]

Indeed, that strong similarities exist in terms of gender dysphoria in these two groups might argue against gender variance as a psychopathology. As a corollary, if each of these sets of clinical conditions constitutes a singular, or at least strongly similar, set of psychosocial developmental difficulties, clinicians might question ascribing a DSM diagnosis to the core features of the conditions.

Children with normal genitalia but who have gender dysphoria—for example, GID—are well-described throughout this issue. But is gender dysphoria the same in children with DSD? As demonstrated later in this discussion, clinical assessments in these conditions might argue for strong similarities. First, in any assessment of children with either of these conditions, one important focus must include considerations of appropriate interventions with respect to any gender variance. Second, to produce a coherent set of diagnostic formulations in either category, there should be some coherence between childhood, adolescent, and even adult formulations in terms of development—typical children, after all, and typical adults do not seek a change from their neonatally assigned sex. But children with gender variance and some with DSD sometimes assert a gender opposite to their assigned sex-of-rearing. Third, treatment considerations might be expected to be similar if the two categories of children bear similar manifestations of gender identity and, perhaps, gender role. In this exploration of child development in children with DSD, perhaps gender dysphoria phenomena can be satisfactorily compared between GID and DSD.

First, however, we must clarify our position regarding the contentious issue of the limits of child development. For our current purposes, in terms of DSD, it is useful to look at development from zygote to birth, in childhood, and subsequently at adolescence and the gradual emergence of adulthood. It is not necessary to establish a predetermined endpoint, because various mechanisms of development remain operative throughout adulthood. Certain points, or limits, of processes must be recognized. Thus, it is conventional to divide development into stages. Divisions of development like the ones previously mentioned are necessarily arbitrary and, when defined in the literature at all, are often prescribed according to rules (such as specific, if somewhat arbitrary, age limits or specific levels of sexual development, ie., Tanner stages) with varying degrees of usefulness. Yet such limits are requirements of scientific discourse. What is crucial is to avoid mistaking the necessities of conceptual speech for discernable events in the development itself; the stages or phases are not discrete phenomena. Development is a continuous, if limited, and unfolding process.

Next, it is important to be clear about what we mean by development in children with DSD. In general, child development involves a series of variably continuous and complex processes and patterns based on genetic makeup, environmental conditions, and the interactions of the two—frequently or constantly interacting. However it is meaningless to speak of development without having in mind that which the development is moving toward; this destination is how we distinguish development from mere change. Thus, the processes in question become intelligible by their intrinsic direction: the development of the embryo is understood with a view to the fetus, and the developing fetus with a view to the child. Interactions between developmental processes occur at every level and are highly complex leaving much room for anomaly, especially in prenatal development. Major prenatal anomalies are often lethal. Lesser anomalies can wreak havoc for parents, physicians, and the postnatal individual. When anomalous genitalia are involved, the newborn typically has normal intelligence, little morbidity, and low mortality. That is, the newborn is otherwise apparently normal.

The critical point is that a child need not be considered a complete or finished individual in order to have an unambiguous identity. On the contrary, the latter (an unambiguous identity) is a necessary condition of the former (a finished individual). Moreover, the manifold aspects of adult identity, cast in social, legal, physiological, and spiritual terms, grow out of the singular sense of identity rooted in the child's self-understanding. But regardless of the relativity of any particular stage of development to certain external cues and model-specific interpretations of those cues, this underlying identity of the child must be considered wholly unique and with sole reference to the individual child in question. The clinician is therefore under an obligation to impose definite standards of care to protect a child's uniqueness and immutability as an individual, not to mention perceiving what that individuality means to the child's identity. Any evaluation or consideration of intervention for a child with atypical sexuality is necessarily an ethical issue and must be treated as such.

Difficulties arise, therefore, at least for the interested adults, when anomalous developments render the external signs of a neonate's sex highly elusive or even misleading. In the mid-20th century, clinicians began using the term *ambiguous genitalia* to indicate phenotypic/genotypic anomalies, especially in terms of genital appearance.[4,5] The term also implies the clinical difficulties of determining an appropriate sex-of-rearing– that is, of the gender the individual would ultimately realize. This difficulty resulted in unsophisticated diagnoses such as female pseudohermaphrodite or true hermaphrodite—with etiological factors not generally considered in diagnoses because they were largely unknown. This lack of sophistication represented the few causative clues clinicians then had—whether the neonate's karyotype was XX or XY or whether the neonate had or had not responded to prenatal androgen exposure.

However, clinical diagnostic sophistication has improved over the decades. In particular, nearly all XX newborns with DSD are found to have a diagnosis of congenital adrenal hyperplasia (CAH). The pathologic origin or causation in these conditions is an adrenal defect in one of a variety of enzymatic pathways. The defects variably retard or prevent the biosynthesis of the normal end products of adrenal steroids, glucocorticoid (cortisol) and mineralocorticoid (a salt-retaining steroid). Both are required for sustaining life. Therefore, the failed synthesis of the required steroids leads to an accumulation of molecular precursors stimulating alternative, minor adrenal biosynthetic pathways. These minor alternative pathways are active in all normal fetuses but with very low-level activity, and they lead to (low-level) androgen production. In CAH, the activity is abnormally high, if variable. Thus, in CAH the adrenal errors commonly lead to prenatal virilization of female genital development. The male fetus is fully virilized already by testicular products or byproducts. Virilization occurs differentially from XX fetus to XX fetus, depending on the specific biosynthetic defect, with the severest virilization occurring in salt-losing forms of CAH. Thus, XX neonates demonstrate inappropriately mild, moderate, or high external genital virilization depending on timing and quantity of the prenatal androgen exposure. These variations in phenotype further complicate assigning a sex-of-rearing.

In the mid-20th century, Money[4] began publishing clinical research on the development of children with DSD (termed *intersex* until recently). Money first reported, in his doctoral dissertation,[5] that as adults, the majority of intersex people identified their gender as their sex assigned at birth. This fact became clinically relevant because advances in reconstructive surgical techniques now allow fairly successful reconstruction of virilized female genitalia, or feminizing genitoplasty. Additionally, XX neonates with CAH had normal internal female genitalia as well as ovaries. Thus, they were not only potentially fertile, but also their genitalia could be feminized surgically. Therefore, XX neonates with CAH have been almost universally assigned to female sex-of-rearing at birth despite the degree of virilization, because they can be feminized surgically, raised female, and can function sexually as female.[5,6]

On the other hand, today we are still able to diagnose only about half of the neonates with an XY DSD—those who have a Y chromosome, or at least the SRY gene from the Y chromosome, the testis-determining gene, or testes-determining factor. These XY neonates with DSD have experienced inadequate (for a male) prenatal androgen effects. Therefore, XY neonates are variably but inadequately virilized at birth, often with a severely inadequate phallus. Despite, or partly because of, surgical advances in feminizing genitoplasty, together with an inability to surgically construct a functional penis, these XY neonates had traditionally also been assigned to a female sex-of-rearing at birth: they could be feminized surgically, raised female, and in adulthood, it was argued, they could perform sexually quite satisfactorily as females. Thus, these children were castrated, even if their testes were normal, and reconstructed with feminizing genitoplasty in early infancy.[7]

The reasoning was simple, if simplistic: if it was until recently nearly impossible to surgically construct a functional penis de novo and if constructing a functional vagina could be successful, and further, if a child (at least a child with a DSD) would self-identify while growing into adulthood with the gender assigned at birth, then newborn boys with an inadequate potential for a functional penis could and should be raised female from birth. There were later reports in the surgical literature of potentially disastrous psychosexual development in such children if they were raised male but without a penis. Clinical decision-makers visualized their role as adopters of a surgical and social paradigm, the "optimal gender policy" —assignment of sex-of-rearing based on the expected optimal outcome in terms of psychosexual, reproductive, and overall development. Being able to perform sexually as a female was thought to be far superior to being unable to perform sexually at all as a male.

The clinical realities and the surgical experiences and realities arising from these early studies were that a large percentage of children with clinically-phenotypically significant DSD, whether XY or XX, were assigned female sex-of-rearing at birth. Socially, surgically, and psychosexually this approach was expected to lead to successful outcomes. Outcomes would include gender identity, gender role, sexual function, sexual satisfaction, and sexual orientation. But outcome data were for a long time curiously lacking.

Thus, the twofold reasoning (1) the potential for fertility (in XX neonates, at least) and potential for functioning genitals, that is, a vagina, and (2) the expected appropriate (for assigned-sex) gender identity outcome along with psychosexual development draws an even more curious inference: (1) that from any neonate a girl can be made or created and that girls will be girls; and (2) that boys are only worthwhile (at least developmentally) if they have a penis, an adequate penis, or a good penis.

Of course, phenotype was partly in the eyes of the beholder: an inadequate penis in one clinic might be deemed adequate in another. Also, would an apparently successful feminizing genitoplasty in the infant render to the adolescent or adult a successful, functioning genital structure leading to sexual satisfaction? This seemingly rhetorical question may in fact have been naive. Indeed, later reports revealed sex function hobbled by introital complications, requiring sometimes-successful surgical re-reconstructions. Even if surgeries were successful, the vagina was satisfactory only for the partner.

Additional difficulties became apparent in brain phenotype. For example, these XX CAH girls' sexual orientation, who they might desire sexual contact with, their desire to carry babies, and so forth—important outcomes of psychosexual development— were unpredictable. This unpredictability was also the case for XY DSD individuals. Whereas specific studies[8-11] addressing these outcomes are too detailed to discuss here, female psychosexual behavioral phenotypes did not necessarily unfold as predicted.

The newborn with an absence of easily identified genitalia is almost always assigned a sex-of-rearing. Again, this assignment remains a clinical conundrum: because the sex of the child is not apparent and because a neonate cannot provide clear communication, a critical sex-of-rearing decision must be made in the neonatal period. This is true socially, legally, psychologically, and especially if the child is to become assimilated to the societal norms of gender identity. Thus, the search for predictive criteria begins, both immediately for the affected newborn and, more generally, in clinical research.

Reductionist approaches to development may offer insight into stages of sex development including gender identity development and sexual orientation. However, such approaches use a degree of precision (determining the child's karyotype, for example) or of construct-formation (social learning or cognitive theories), which can easily obscure the global phenomena, especially for the newborn. Such approaches risk missing the real forest for the assumed trees. But in any clinical situation, regardless of the particular complications at issue, it is the whole human being who is being treated. This is important to recognize given the delicate nature of children's attachment to their genitalia, their genital abnormality perhaps being too often communicated in the child's clinical exposures. Additionally, the relationship between genitalia and identity cannot be ignored: fertility (long-term, of course) and pleasure (short-term and long-term).[4] The effects of clinical approaches on the overall development of these children and their long-term functionality as adults can be substantial, and the gravity of their situation demands clinical prudence.

As a testimony to experience in clinical approaches, we would cite the senior author's (W.G.R.'s) work in the SUCCEED clinic at the University of Oklahoma Health Sciences Center, a growing multidisciplinary clinic for the assessment and treatment of children, adolescents, and adults with DSD (see www.succeedclinic.org).[12] (SUCCEED is a designation intended to avoid any negative connotations.) The clinic currently follows about 50 children with XX and about 50 with XY DSD. Additionally, the senior author (W.G.R.) also has had clinical experience with over 200 children with major urogenital anomalies, mostly the exstrophy-epispadias complex (ie, epispadias, classical bladder exstrophy, or cloacal exstrophy) and about 100 children with DSD who would have formerly been termed *intersex*.[13,14] As a group, these children exhibit a variety of personalities, cognitive skill sets, temperaments, and other dimensional qualities. They also come from a range of socioeconomic backgrounds and have a range of clinical histories. However, all of these children have a DSD, and more than 150 are XY individuals assigned female sex-of-rearing as a neonate.[10,11,13]

DEVELOPMENTAL PSYCHOPATHOLOGY IN CHILDREN WITH DSD

How does an assessment of psychopathology inform our understanding of child development in DSD? First, developmental psychopathology is a relatively recent extension and amalgam of multiple disciplines in pediatric psychology and psychiatry that consider psychopathologic conditions in and from childhood.[15] Like normal development, psychopathologic conditions develop within complex genetic and environmental processes and their interactions and as they supervene on preexisting development and preexisting psychopathologic conditions. It is beyond the scope of this article to elaborate, but we must have recourse to the notion of developmental psychopathology to pose the guiding question of this *Clinics* issue.

Simplistically, there may be two common issues of developmental psychopathology in children with DSD who have gender issues: internalizing disorders such as anxiety and depressive disorders, and gender dysphoria with problems related to sex reassignment. First, many of these children seem to have problems of internalizing disorders, presumably from multiple causative factors, but usually not of externalizing disorders. As in gender-variant (non-DSD) children, internalizing disorders frequently appear in childhood or adolescence, can be fleeting or long-term, and have the potential to transform into disorders in adulthood.

Within the purview of developmental psychopathology, do the core features of gender dysphoria fit, whether in children with DSD or GID? First, clinical experience with children with DSD reveals that gender dysphoria might be more accurately described as discordant recognition of sex-of-self from sex-of-rearing, which might seem not unlike children with GID. Children with DSD who are misassigned in the neonatal period and who come to recognize such misassignment are not so much dysphoric about their assigned sex as they are cognizant. They develop a growing awareness that their sex-of-rearing is discordant with their developing perceptions. For some of these children, their later unfolding recognition of sexual orientation strongly influences this perception of discordance.

Children with GID may be upset with their assigned sex, or they may say that they are sad because they want to be the opposite sex. They may hate their genitalia and only grudgingly accept that their "real" sex is the one assigned neonatally. In contradistinction to this mindset, children with DSD tend to be more accepting of their assigned sex but recognize that it is simply incorrect or that it was incorrectly assigned. They do not typically hate their genitalia (however unusual in appearance), and often they can calmly entertain the notion that they are or might be one sex or the other, whether or not they feel that such assignment is appropriate. As adolescents, these children may deny, to their parents, for example, that they are homosexual, despite being attracted to a person of the same sex because they do not regard their sex-of-rearing as their true sex. In other words, they do not reject homosexuality per se; rather, they deny the authenticity of their sex-of-rearing.[11,13] It must be recognized that children with DSD dichotomize. They see themselves, and presumably others, as either male or female, heterosexual or homosexual; neither attribution is particularly troubling to them in itself. But these children are signally concerned with receiving from others the "correct" attribution for themselves. Indeed, it is fascinating that many of these children do not describe internal aspects of gender dysphoria, as seems to be more typical of children with GID. Rather, if children with DSD have any strong discordant feelings, they more commonly recognize that an error has been made, that they are in fact the opposite sex. They do not reject their assigned sex as such; they reject the authenticity of it. This recognition, if and when it occurs in a child with a particular DSD, is more likely to occur in children between 4 and 9 years of age or around or after puberty, but it can also occur into their 20s.[13,16] Postpubescents and people in their mid-20s with gender dysphoria may or may not have had strong doubts about their sex-of-rearing as children. But when they recognize their sexual orientation, and as they work and live socially, they "find themselves": they recognize their gender role, their attitudes, their interests and their sexual orientation as an of internal combination that must constitute a being of the opposite sex. This recognition represents their internal full evidence, that their true sex is opposite to their sex-of-rearing.

The literature on adolescents with the following conditions seems to demonstrate this recognition well: (1) 5α-reductase-2 deficiency,[8] (2) cloacal exstrophy,[11] and (3) some cases of mosaic 46,XY/45,X-.[11,13] With these conditions one of the following holds true: (1) testosterone (T) effects are normal, although T cannot be metabolized into the more potent androgen dihydrotestosterone (DHT) because of a genetic enzymatic defect, 5α-reductase-2 deficiency; DHT is required in order to virilize the external genitalia, but not the brain so that these XY neonates look female at birth, albeit with normal (undescended) testes; or (2) T effects and DHT effects are normal but a major fetal tissue error leads to an absent penis (cloacal exstrophy); or, (3) T effects are high enough to virilize the brain but not high enough to lead to adequate DHT levels to fully virilize the genitalia (mosaic XY/X-).

In contrast, there is a distinct absence of such discordance in children with complete androgen insensitivity syndrome, also known as testicular feminization. With this condition, normal testes lead to normal end products, but there is an absence of the androgen receptor molecule: androgens have no effect at all. These XY individuals are raised female and see themselves as female.[17]

CLINICAL MEDICAL APPROACHES TO CHILDREN WITH DSD

Outcomes with DSD have pointed to a lack of understanding of much of gender identity development. First, DSD have a rather unique clinical history from the mid-20th century to the present, as evident in the literature. The origins of this history lie in the clinical recognition that abnormal genitalia could in some instances be reconstructed.[7] However, this recognition applied to female genital reconstruction only. The enormous difficulties in constructing a functional penis rendered those attempts fruitless.[10,11] Such endeavors were considered impossible from the point of view of adequate sexual functioning.

Over the course of the 20th century, the idea of determinative significance of the genitalia for gender identity development, increasingly upheld by psychological and psychoanalytic ideas, gave rise to a moral imperative to "build" genitalia for children who seemed otherwise sexually doomed by their developmental disorders. This imperative, added to the accepted importance of sexual functioning, evolved into the clinical-surgical paradigm of assigning neonatal sex as female.[7]

GENDER IDENTITY, CLINICAL PRUDENCE, AND ETHICAL QUESTIONS

Despite the seeming diversity of children with DSD and GID, certain developmental vulnerabilities have remained constant. Some early exposures, some early experiences, and some unknown combination of these play a role in the determination of developmental vulnerabilities, how they are expressed, and what outcomes might be expected. We know of only a few constitutional parameters that are likely to predominate (eg, high prenatal androgen levels) but little is known about how or how much or which environmental parameters might moderate or mediate the outcomes for a given trait or behavioral phenotype (eg, how varying levels of androgen interact differentially with specific genes). Also, it is unclear how specific combinations of factors might be especially important to some children. We do know that prenatal exposure to effective androgen seems to be strongly associated with male-typical behaviors in a dose-response relationship. We know that androgen exposure also seems to be associated with a propensity toward sexual attraction to females. We know little about mechanisms, however, and whether or how these associations might be causal. If mechanisms are deterministic, even if only partially, it is unclear as well why prenatal exposure to androgen is associated with sexual attraction to males rather than to females in some individuals. Causative factors in sexual orientation have complex patterns of interactions.

From a research standpoint, gender identity is even more difficult to predict. The precise mechanisms of gender identity development are complex, the interactions of the mechanisms poorly understood, and the outcomes not entirely clear, except that children and adolescents nearly always dichotomize. (For an excellent review of gene and environment interactions in gender identity development along with theoretical underpinnings, see the review by Ruble and colleagues.[18]) Unfortunately, gene-environment interactions are poorly understood. Indeed, even something as seemingly simple as height, for example, reveals that hundreds or thousands of gene polymorphisms interacting with a multitude of environmental factors affect the outcome, each with a small effect.[19] Something as complex as who we are or how we express who we are would be expected to be far more difficult to explain, and may have no finite or endpoint parameters. Gene-environment interactions may be additive, multiplicative, or mixed, depending on many other factors.

Confounding studies even further, early experiences have complex interactions in child development. Children with DSD have variably distinctive early experiences including anesthetics, surgeries, and multiple medical visits. How these experiences interact with or effect changes in the developing brain, such as alterations in the developing hypothalamic-pituitary-adrenal axis, is unclear. Behavioral manifestations might also be related to perceived reactions of parents, implications for urinary and sexual function, and body and genital image issues that may arise during development. The authors stress that the genetic and environmental actions and interactions cannot be ignored; however, they also suggest that in assessing these children's own sense of gender, within their own sense of identity, we must ultimately rely on them.

ETHICAL ASPECTS OF NORMALIZING CHILDREN

The question of gender dysphoria as a symptom of psychopathologic conditions in children with DSD, therefore, would seem to be different from gender dysphoria in children with GID. However, these two conditions may have much in common. We can ask, for example, How are parental responses related between the groups? What are the effects of the differences in early experiences? What are the effects of clinical responses? These considerations are even more important when parents and clinicians entertain medical interventions.

There seems to be a contemporary need to normalize children with DSD and to acquiesce to the desires of children with GID. This trend may be traced to the more fundamental human need, frequently expressed by children themselves, to be "normal." To say that man is a social animal is to say that human beings naturally desire to fit in with similar people. This desire survives, ironically, in a universal encomium to individuality and "individual difference." We speak to a child of the importance of "being yourself" when the need to be accepted into the group is the issue (ie, when being like others is the goal). The problem later becomes obscure for adults, who believe that subtle variations constitute different choices or indicate diversity. In this case the truth proceeds "from the mouths of babes," who generally detest what is different from everybody else, especially in themselves. It is natural for children to want to be like others, to be a member of a group, to be normal.[20]

In the context of children with DSD GID, normalizing has surgical, psychological, and hormonal consequences.[21] This normalizing is a great controversy, and perhaps the only assertion that can be made with clinical solvency seems more like a disclaimer: There is no universally successful approach. Nevertheless, we do not oppose the suggestion that surgical or medical normalization of children with DSD or GID might be important developmentally; it certainly can be important functionally. We also do not deny that the prevention of later need/desire for sex reassignment might be beneficial in the long term for some children with GID. However, in both conditions these approaches should be contextualized. Our efforts to help these children to fit in "like everybody else" must be coordinated with a sense of the uniqueness of each child, or with a constant view to how each child is unlike anybody else.

Particular approaches must involve a certain degree of latitude to accommodate unanticipated variations of human behavior or reactivity that we have come to expect in the field. Naturally, this does not mean that every concern or desire of parents or children should be gratified, even if, or especially when, we understand or sympathize with them. We must be flexible in the face of changing circumstances without losing sight of the long-term outcomes for these children, considered individually and as their outcomes aggregate or diverge nosologically. Strictly speaking, the legitimacy of any approach is determined by outcomes, and therefore by the children themselves, or rather by what the children consider retrospectively as adolescents or adults. The situation could seem to put additional burden on the clinician of becoming a prophet. Unfortunately, such a retrospective qualification is a reality for all clinicians who concern themselves with gender dysphoria and DSD. Child development refuses to be an exact science. It is with seasoned modesty that we emphasize, to different degrees, the changeability of children during growth and development.

This changeability is the case in children with either DSD or GID. Gender dysphoria, however, as discussed earlier, seems to be distinct in children with GID. Children with DSD seem to portray less cognitive rigidity, less attachment to a gender. In other words, these children—despite whether parents or clinicians hold rigidly to the child being one gender or the other—seem to have more openness to the idea of what gender they are or should be than children with GID. They can typically discuss being one gender or the other with less emotional baggage.

On the other hand, in children with DSD or GID, it is the sense of self-recognition as a gender that seems to be fundamental within the child's brain that stands out phenomenologically. In either DSD or GID, however, the child (or the parent) is seeking who or what the child is. This similarity may be paramount.

THE IMPERATIVE OF THE ETHICAL DISCUSSION

Scientific research today sometimes betrays the seeming naiveté of questions that result from a lack of familiarity with the natural hierarchy of problems or with what philosophers refer to as ethics. With regard to current discussions of normalizing children, researchers frequently mistake the axiomatic for the problematic; that is, they bring into question what are in fact the conditions of any questions. Thus it is inquired whether children desire, and their parents desire them, to be, "normal," when in fact the answer to this question is the specific condition for their seeking clinical help. Science is constitutionally unable to persuade people who are suffering that they are OK, making it incumbent on the clinician to alleviate their suffering in whatever way he or she sees fit. The ethical conundrum around the question of whose suffering ultimately determines the treatment: that of the parents or that of the children, or even that of the clinician? Whose expectations are decisive when it comes to what is normal for the child? As any experienced clinician would admit, these are tantalizing questions that arise again and again. And it is precisely this character of the questions that determines them as genuine questions of ethics.

Ethical questions may be distinguished from scientific questions on the basis of their content: they are concerned with the proper or "right" course of action. It is the prerogative of the clinician as a competent judge of the field to decide what is ethical. The clinician as scientist, in contrast, is concerned with what is merely necessary, given the proper course of action. It is the essence of the ethical to defy formulation or reduction to universal rules, the magnanimous efforts of the greatest minds notwithstanding. There is no substitute for clinical prudence and good judgment. Accordingly, it is our duty as clinicians to be familiar with the nature of the problem and the parties involved.

Yet the situation with which we are concerned is not only frustrated by the potentially conflicting desires among parents, children, and physicians at any given phase of intervention. Clinicians who undertake to treat these children must also vie with conflicting desires within the same individuals over time—that is, mere change. Our aim is to foster normal child development, and what children desire of themselves as children is rarely what satisfies them as adults. We naturally defer to the desires of the parents in such matters. However, a substantial part of normal development involves the child making independent self-assessments and transforming these into honest communication, regardless of the opinions or reactions of adults. Therefore, the child must be allowed to contradict the parents, sometimes radically, before any decision is made. This requirement means the clinician must resist the temptation to play the soothsayer to the parents or otherwise to prevent "waves"; the integrity of a clinical evaluation demands it. Yet perhaps it is safest to give precedence to the opinions of parents. Problems of this sort are at the heart of any honest, sustained, and deliberate discussion of what we call intersex ethics—a discussion we must consistently promote, or at any rate, one that we cannot honestly avoid.

SUMMARY

We must at this time resist both concrete conclusions and ethereal musings. Nevertheless, longitudinally following children with DSD—a large and diverse group—may help us in potent ways to understand the evolving sense of self as one sex or the other. This group of individuals would seem very different generally, and even more specifically, to those anatomically normal children with gender dysphoria. This latter group would seem less diverse behaviorally, cognitively, and emotionally, at least in terms of gender identity.

Still, there is important concordance in the mechanisms of children of either group, those with DSD or those with GID, expressing their gender identity. In their affirmation of their internally recognized identity, those children who express strong gender dysphoria are phenomenologically strikingly similar.

Whatever their similarities and differences, the two groups of children provide us with an emphasis on recognizing the importance of the individual and the individual's long-term, developmental well-being when we make clinical decisions that involve intervening in their lives or bodies. They probably also emphasize how important it is or ought to be that we do not intervene in any way that cannot be undone if the growing child, adolescent, or emerging adult so sees himself or herself to have changed as opposed to developed.

REFERENCES

1. Houk CP, Hughes IA, Ahmed SF, et al. Summary of consensus statement on intersex disorders and their management. International Intersex Consensus Conference. Pediatrics 2006;118(2):753–7.
2. American Psychological Association. DSM-5; the future of psychiatric diagnosis. DSM-5 development. Available at: http://www.dsm5.org. Accessed August 20, 2011.
3. Meyer-Bahlburg HF. From mental disorder to iatrogenic hypogonadism: dilemmas in conceptualizing gender identity variants as psychiatric conditions. Arch Sex Behav 2010;39(2):461–76.
4. Money J. Sex errors of the body and related syndromes. Baltimore (MD): Paul H. Brooks; 1994. p. 1–6, 60–84, 108–9.
5. Money JW. Hermaphroditism, an inquiry into the nature of a human paradox[dissertation]. Cambridge (MA): Harvard University; 1952.
6. Hughes IA, Houk C, Ahmed SF, et al. Consensus statement on management of intersex disorders. Arch Dis Child 2006;91(7):554–63.
7. Glassberg KI. The intersex infant: early gender assignment and surgical reconstruction. J Pediatr Adolesc Gynecol 1998;11(3):151–4.
8. Imperato-McGinley J, Peterson RE, Gautier T, et al. Androgens and the evolution of male-gender identity among male pseudohermaphrodites with 5alpha-reductase deficiency. N Engl J Med 1979;300(22):1233–7.
9. Reiner WG, Kropp BP. A 7-year experience of genetic males with severe phallic inadequacy assigned female. J Urol 2004;172(6 pt 1):2395–8 [discussion: 2398].
10. Reiner WG, Gearhart JP. Discordant sexual identity in some genetic males with cloacal exstrophy assigned to female sex at birth. N Engl J Med 2004;350(4):333–41.
11. Reiner WG. Psychosexual development in genetic males assigned female: the cloacal exstrophy experience. Child Adolesc Psychiatr Clin N Am 2004;13(3):657–74, ix.
12. Schaeffer TL, Tryggestad JB, Mallappa A, et al. An evidence-based model of multidisciplinary care for patients and families affected by classical congenital adrenal hyperplasia due to 21-hydroxylase deficiency. Int J Pediatr Endocrinol 2010;2010:692439.
13. Reiner WG. Gender identity and sex-of-rearing in children with disorders of sexual differentiation. J Pediatr Endocrinol Metab 2005;18(6):549–53.

14. Reiner W. Developmental perspectives of children with genitourinary anomalies. In: Gearhart J, Rink RC, Mouriquand P, editors. Pediatric Urology. 2nd edition. Philadelphia: Saunders; 2010. p. 267–79.
15. Rutter M. Developmental psychopathology as a research perspective. In: Magnusson D, Casaer PJM, editors. Longitudinal research on individual development: present status and future perspectives. New York: Cambridge University Press; 1993. p. 127–52.
16. Meyer-Bahlburg HF. Male gender identity in an XX individual with congenital adrenal hyperplasia. J Sex Med 2009;6(1):297–8 [author reply: 298–9].
17. Mazur T. Gender dysphoria and gender change in androgen insensitivity or micropenis. Arch Sex Behav 2005;34(4):411–21.
18. Ruble DN, Martin CL, Berenbaum SA. Gender development. In: Eisenberg N, editor. Handbook of child psychology, vol. 3. 6th edition. Hoboken (NJ): John Wiley and Sons, Inc; 2006. p. 858–932.
19. Lango Allen H, Estrada K, Lettre G, et al. Hundreds of variants clustered in genomic loci and biological pathways affect human height. Nature 2010;467(7317):832–8.
20. Gooren L. Foreword to the second edition. In: Money J, editor. Sex errors of the body and related syndromes. 2nd edition. Baltimore (MD): Paul H. Brookes Publishing Co; 1994. p. ix–xii.
21. Parens E, editor. Surgically shaping children: technology, ethics, and the pursuit of normality. Baltimore (MD): Johns Hopkins University Press; 2006.

Gender Monitoring and Gender Reassignment of Children and Adolescents with a Somatic Disorder of Sex Development

Heino F.L. Meyer-Bahlburg, Dr rer nat

KEYWORDS

- Disorders of sex development • Gender identity
- Gender reassignment • Intersexuality

The term *disorder of sex development* (DSD) refers to somatic conditions of atypical development of the reproductive tract.[1] It includes the conditions traditionally denoted as intersexuality. In intersexuality, certain primary genetic factors of sexual determination (ie, those regulating the gonadal differentiation into testes or ovaries and/or certain primary genetic and hormonal factors of sexual differentiation of the reproductive tract [that presumably also affect the brain]) are in some way dysfunctional.[2] Examples of classical intersexuality are such syndromes as 46,XX congenital adrenal hyperplasia (CAH); 46,XY androgen insensitivity; or 46,XY 5α-reductase-2 deficiency (5α-R2-D). DSD includes, in addition, syndromes or conditions involving genital abnormalities that are caused by other developmental factors (eg, cloacal exstrophy of the bladder, penile agenesis, or vaginal agenesis).[1] If at birth the external genitalia look ambiguous, in other words not clearly male or female, or if upon more detailed medical examinations and tests the reproductive tract as a whole seems to deviate from the normative male or female pattern, gender assignment may not be straightforward and based on the appearance of the externa genitalia. Instead, it may require the establishment of a medical diagnosis and its degree of severity as well as a consideration of the impact of the atypical etiologic factors on the sexual differentiation of the brain and later behavior and, thereby, on the long-term gender outcome as supported by empirical evidence.

Gender assignment guidelines in such cases have varied considerably across historical eras and diverse cultures.[3] Yet even at the current status of such policies,[1]

The author has nothing to disclose.

New York State Psychiatric Institute, Department of Psychiatry, Columbia University, 1051 Riverside Drive, Unit 15, New York, NY 10032, USA

E-mail address: meyerb@childpsych.columbia.edu

Child Adolesc Psychiatric Clin N Am 20 (2011) 639–649

doi:10.1016/j.chc.2011.07.002

childpsych.theclinics.com

Table 1
Rates of patient-initiated gender change (or marked gender dysphoria) in published cases

DSD Syndrome	Female to Male (%)	Male to Female (%)
46,XX Congenital adrenal hyperplasia[5]	5.2	12.1
46,XY 5α-reductase 2 deficiency[6]	63.0–66.0	0.0
46,XY 17β-hydroxysteroid dehydrogenase 3 deficiency[6]	64.0	0.0
46,XY Complete androgen insensitivity[7]	0.0	—
46,XY Partial androgen insensitivity[7]	7.0	14.0
46,XY micropenis[7]	0.0	3.0
46,XY nonhormonal DSD[8]	35.0	0.3

long-term follow-up data are limited, and with it prognostic accuracy as to long-term outcome in terms of gender identity, sexual functioning, and related aspects of the general quality of life. Available data show that the rates of later gender dysphoria and/or patient-initiated gender change vary considerably, from zero to about two-thirds of patients, across syndromes, with syndrome severity, and with initial gender assignment (**Table 1**).[4–8] These data indicate that, overall, the rate of gender dysphoria and patient-initiated gender change is considerably higher among individuals with marked genital ambiguity than the rate of transsexualism in the general (non-DSD) population.[9] Therefore, clinicians who provide services for persons with serious problems of gender identity are likely to encounter some individuals with a DSD among their clients and need to be familiar with their specific presentations and problems, unless they refer such patients to other providers with special expertise in DSD-related gender problems.

Given the differences in presentation and context of gender dysphoria and patient-initiated gender change in patients with a DSD[10] and the fact that the hormonal abnormality in such cases provides a plausible explanation for the atypical gender development, the *Diagnostic and Statistical Manual of Mental Disorders,* 4th edition, treatment revision (DSM-IV-TR) of the American Psychiatric Association[11] excluded patients with DSD from the diagnosis of gender identity disorder (GID), even if they met the behavioral criteria for GID. A possible revision of this policy is under consideration for the next edition, DSM-5, expected in 2013 (see www.dsm5.org).

We know from clinical experience that later change of gender is associated with significant emotional, social, and financial burdens, although these have not yet been studied systematically. Moreover, such gender change may be further complicated when it has been preceded by surgical and hormonal treatments in line with the originally assigned gender. These considerations imply that formulations of policies of DSD management designed to minimize the likelihood of later gender change should include the following[12]: (1) the gender assigned at birth should be chosen so as to minimize the risk of later gender change; (2) gender-confirming genital surgery should be performed only if the long-term prognosis for maintenance of the assigned gender is based on reasonably solid evidence, which requires a definitive genetic/endocrine diagnosis and clear ascertainment of its severity, along with acceptable data on the long-term gender outcome of individuals of that category of diagnosis and severity; (3) gender reassignment, if justified by satisfactory evidence, should be done relatively early in development so as to prevent later medical treatments that would be at odds with a possible later gender change.

REFERRAL CONTEXT

A variety of circumstances may prompt a reconsideration of the original gender assignment and, if the child is old enough, a comprehensive evaluation of his/her gender development. Referral to a more specialized medical setting may lead to a change or refinement of the genetic and/or endocrine diagnosis, which may imply a different prognosis for long-term gender outcome. Different physicians may differ in the conclusions they draw from the degree of genital ambiguity for the prognosis of gender development and outcome of genital surgery for a boy versus a girl. In the author's experience, such conclusion may be made when a child with DSD is referred to a surgeon for "corrective" surgery designed to bring the appearance of the genitalia in line with the assigned gender, thereby "confirming" the assigned gender. In late childhood or early adolescence, children with a variety of DSD syndromes may develop unexpected secondary sex characteristics, for instance, breasts in a 46,XX child with Prader-5 CAH assigned to the male gender or overall virilizing puberty in a 46,XY child with 5α-R2-D growing up prepubertally as a girl. An endocrinologist may feel uneasy inducing female puberty by hormone-replacement therapy in a 46,XY child who had been assigned female and gonadectomized in infancy but now shows strongly masculinized gender-related behavior. Some children or adolescents with DSD and markedly gender-atypical behavior may become uncertain which gender they really belong to and, may feel confused about it or even develop gender dysphoria and the desire to change their gender.

AGE AT GENDER REASSIGNMENT

At what age should gender reassignment be done, if indicated? The answer needs to be informed by what is known about normative early gender development,[13,14] although what is typical is only partially understood. Cognitively normal infants begin to categorize other people by gender in infancy. During the second year of life, gendered toy and game preferences emerge. By the time of their third birthday, most children classify themselves consistently as boy or girl. Such developmental data imply that 18 months as the upper limit for imposing gender reassignment, which was proposed at much earlier stages of our knowledge of gender development[15] was not based on satisfactory data and may have to be lowered.

Such considerations are reflected in recommendations that have recently emerged for gender reassignment in children with DSD.[1,16] In infancy, gender reassignment can proceed without psychological evaluation of the child if well-justified by correct DSD diagnosis and findings from long-term outcome studies, and if genuinely supported by the parents. However, once the child is mature enough for psychological gender assessment, gender reassignment must be based on a thorough psychological gender evaluation. In the author's opinion, therefore, gender-confirming genital surgery should be delayed, especially in female-assigned 46,XY cases with likely prenatal androgen exposure above that expected for endocrinologically normal females, until a stable gender identity appears to have been established. Exceptions have to be made when there are strong contraindications such as age-inappropriate enuresis, urinary tract infections explainable by anatomic problems, or unalterable, strong, harmful social stigma related to obvious genital ambiguity.

EVALUATION FOR GENDER REASSIGNMENT

Gender reassignment may imply major changes—legal, social, often somatic—for the patient. It may also profoundly affect the patient's family. Parents lose a child of one gender, which may be deeply felt, and need to adjust to having a child of another gender instead. Similarly, siblings lose a brother or a sister. The neighbors may question the decision or form adverse opinions about the patient's family. Institutions such as religious communities and schools may need to be persuaded to accept the patient in his/her new gender role. For adolescent and adult patients, gender change may have marked consequences for their standing among their peers and their romantic or marital relationships, and they may need to negotiate the transition with supervisors and colleagues at their place of work. Thus, a decision on gender reassignment must be based on a solid and comprehensive evaluation of all domains that are pertinent to the reassignment decision.

The evaluation for gender reassignment includes a careful review of the patient's DSD diagnosis (including its severity) and his/her medical history of hormone treatments and genital operations, pubertal history if applicable, along with a review of the evidence-based prognosis for future endocrine and surgical treatment options, gender development, sexual functioning, and implications for parenthood (including the option of preservation of sperm and ova, if applicable). Further, the evaluation needs to include the gender history such as birth, the events that led to the original gender assignment and the parents' reactions and coping during that time, the development of gender-related behavior and of gender identity including periods of gender uncertainty, gender dysphoria, and prior changes of gender, if any, be they imposed by physicians or parents or initiated by the patient. The clinician should also assess the family's cultural/religious background and embeddedness regarding gender ideology and the associated degree of gender-conforming pressures and societal (and legal) tolerance of gender change (which depends to some extent on the presence of a documentable medical basis for gender change). For instance, many cultures in the Middle East and Far East favor male over female offspring, and sex assignments in newborns with genital ambiguity may be biased accordingly.[17,18] In older patients, the development of sexual orientation, romantic/erotic relationships, and sexual functioning is also of interest, along with an assessment of the patient's current status in these domains, the role of cultural context, and the family's reaction. In addition, the clinician needs to assess the general psychiatric, cognitive, educational, and work history of the patient and his/her quality of life to the extent it is applicable; obtain an overview of the psychosocial outcome of other family members, if any, with the same DSD condition,; and consider other major pertinent aspects of the family's history.

In order to minimize self-presentation biases and to maximize the validity of the evaluation, a multiinformant, multimethod approach should be used. The details will vary, of course, with the age of the patient. In young children, the informants will usually be the parents, the child himself/herself, and occasionally another caretaker who spends considerable amounts of time with the child. In adolescents and adults, especially when one or both parents may not be part of the family any more, other family members who know the patient well may participate, and long-term romantic/sexual partners and spouses may be important sources of information. Also, involvement of school personnel should be considered, albeit with caution. On the one hand, teachers may observe many important aspects of the child's gender presentation in play activities (eg, dress-up corners) and peer relationships. On the other hand, there is always a risk of inappropriate curiosity and stigmatization when the attention of school personnel is directed toward gender-atypical somatic and/or behavioral characteristics.

Systematic methods for the assessment of psychological sex differences in behavior have been developed since at least the 1930s, and recent decades have

Table 2 Assessment domain, title/content, and mode—preschool age		
Domain	**Full Title (or content)**	**Mode**
Parents		
Gender history	(Child's original gender assignment, genital surgery, gender development)	Clinical interview
Psychiatric problems	Child Behavior Checklist for Ages 1 1/2-5[20]	Questionnaire
Gendered behavior	Pre-School Activities Inventory[21]	Questionnaire
Gendered behavior, gender identity, gender dysphoria	Mother form of the Gender-Role Assessment Schedule—Child[a,22]	Semistructured interview
Child Patient		
Psychiatric problems	(Mental status as appropriate for cognitive level)	Clinical interview and observation
Gendered behavior	Play Observation 1 (toys)[23]	Observation
Gendered behavior	Play Observation 2 (dress-up)	Observation
Gender identity	Draw-A-Person Test (modified, with inquiry)[24]	Observation with semistructured interview
Gender identity, gender dysphoria	Gender Identity Interview[25]	Semistructured interview

[a] Mother form of Gender-Role Assessment Schedule–Child. 1982-2 edition. (H.F.L. Meyer-Bahlburg, A.A. Ehrhardt, unpublished manuscript, 1982, available from the first author).

seen the gradual accumulation of assessment methods specifically designed for research and clinical use in patients of different age groups with suspected GID, regardless of the presence or absence of a DSD.[19] Such methods have been devised for reports by parents and others about patients as well as for patients' self-report and for behavior observation of patients by clinicians. Given the small number of clinics specialized in providing services to gender-dysphoric patients, it is no wonder that a formal consensus on a battery of standard assessment tools does not exist. As an illustration, **Tables 2** to **4** list the relatively standardized tool set that the author uses in clinical work. Apart from screening questionnaires for problem behaviors, most of the various age-specific questionnaires and interview schedules are designed to assess various aspects of gendered behavior and gender identity. Given the few behavioral specialists in this area and the logistical problems and costs associated with research on rare disorders, it is not surprising that none of the gender tools use national norms; instead, most rely on comparison values based on reasonable local convenience samples of non-DSD individuals with or without GID, and some are used only qualitatively. For a standard gender evaluation of a new patient, the author plans two sessions with the parents (and/or other informants), two sessions with the patient, and one session for feedback to the parents and/or the patient, each session at 1 1/2 to 2 hours. Occasionally, if there are significant psychiatric problems apart from gender, additional time may have to be scheduled for the evaluation of those. The tool set may be abbreviated for patients who are being seen annually for gender monitoring.

Table 3
Assessment domain, title/content, and mode—middle childhood

Domain	Full Title (or content)	Mode
Parents		
Gender history	(Child's original gender assignment, genital surgery, gender development)	Clinical interview
Psychiatric problems	Child Behavior Checklist for Ages 6–18[26]	Questionnaire
Gendered behavior	Child Game Participation Questionnaire[27]	Questionnaire
Gendered behavior	Child Behavior and Attitude Questionnaire[28]	Questionnaire
Gendered behavior	Gender Identity Questionnaire— Parent[29]	Questionnaire
Gendered behavior, gender identity, gender dysphoria	Mother form of the Gender-Role Assessment Schedule—Child[a,22]	Semistructured interview
Child Patient		
Gender history	(Child's knowledge and experience of gender assignment history and genital surgery, if old enough and informed about this)	Clinical interview
Psychiatric problems	Mental status exam as appropriate for cognitive level	Clinical interview and observation
Gendered behavior	Gender-Role Assessment Schedule—Child[b]	Semistructured interview
Gendered behavior	Play Observation 1 (toys)[23]	Observation
Gendered behavior	Play Observation 2 (dress-up)	Observation
Gender identity	Draw-A-Person Test (modified, with inquiry)[24]	Observation with semistructured interview
Gender identity, gender dysphoria	Gender Identity Interview[25]	Semistructured interview

[a] Mother form of Gender-Role Assessment Schedule–Child (M-GRAS-C). 1982-2 edition. (H.F.L. Meyer-Bahlburg, A.A. Ehrhardt, unpublished manuscript, 1982, available from the first author).
[b] Gender-Role Assessment Schedule–Child (GRAS-C). 1988-2 edition. (H.F.L. Meyer-Bahlburg, A.A. Ehrhardt, unpublished manuscript, 1988, available from the first author).

DECISION ON GENDER REASSIGNMENT AND ITS IMPLEMENTATION

No criteria have been developed specifically for decisions on gender reassignment of children with a DSD and gender dysphoria. Nevertheless, some general recommendations have been formulated by the most recent international consensus conference on DSD[1]: (1) gender-atypical behavior is more common in individuals with a somatic DSD than in the general population, but such behavior by itself should not be taken as an indicator for gender reassignment; (2) in DSD-affected individuals who report significant gender dysphoria, a comprehensive psychological evaluation and an opportunity to explore feelings about gender with a qualified clinician are required over a period of time; (3) if the desire to change gender persists, the patient's wish

Table 4
Assessment domain, title/content, and mode—adolescence and adulthood

Domain	Full Title (or content)	Mode
Parents (and other informants)		
Gender history	(Patient's original gender assignment, genital surgery, gender development)	Clinical interview
Psychiatric problems	Child Behavior Checklist for Ages 6–18[26]	Questionnaire
Gendered behavior	Gender Identity Questionnaire—Parent[29]	Questionnaire
Gendered behavior, gender identity, gender dysphoria	Mother form of the Gender-Role Assessment Schedule – Adolescent and Adult[a]	Semi-structured interview
Adolescent or Adult Patient		
Gender history	(Patient's knowledge and experience of gender assignment history and genital surgery, if old enough and informed about this)	Clinical interview
Psychiatric problems	Youth Self Report[30]	Questionnaire
Psychiatric problems	Mental status exam	Clinical interview and observation
Gendered behavior	Hobby Preferences (modified)[31,32]	Questionnaire
Gendered behavior	Career Questionnaire[32,33]	Questionnaire
Gendered behavior	Recalled Childhood Gender Questionnaire, Revised[34]	Questionnaire
Gendered behavior	Pregnancy and Infant Orientation Questionnaire[35]	Questionnaire
Gendered behavior, gender identity, gender dysphoria	Gender-Role Assessment Schedule—Adolescent or Adult[b]	Semistructured interview
Gender identity, gender dysphoria	Gender Identity/Gender Dysphoria Questionnaire for Adolescents and Adults[36,37]	Questionnaire
Sexual history and current status	Sexual Behavior Assessment Schedule—Adolescents, Adults (section selected according to age and sexual experience)[c]	Semistructured interview

[a] Gender-Role Assessment Schedule–Adult (GRAS-A). 1984 edition. (A.A. Ehrhardt, H.F.L. Meyer-Bahlburg, unpublished manuscript, 1984, available from the second author).
[b] Gender-Role Assessment Schedule–Adult (GRAS-A). 1984 edition. (A.A. Ehrhardt, H.F.L. Meyer-Bahlburg, uunpublished manuscript, 1984, available from the second author).
[c] Sexual Behavior Assessment Schedule–Adult (SEBAS-A). 1983 edition. (H.F.L. Meyer-Bahlburg, A.A. Ehrhardt, unpublished manuscript, 1983, available from the first author).

should be supported and may require the input of a specialist skilled in the management of gender change.

It is important to keep in mind that transient periods of uncertainty about one's gender are common in patients with a DSD but should not be interpreted as a clear indication for gender reassignment. For instance, in a follow-up study of adult 46,XY patients with a DSD, about one-third reported retrospectively that they had experienced a time when they felt unsure about their gender, but most were satisfied with their gender at the time of evaluation.[22] From clinical experience we know that gender uncertainty may arise from such factors as gender-atypical behavior and interests, atypical somatic developments and their social repercussions, and learning about one's gender-atypical medical history or chromosomal status. Supportive counseling and contact with support groups often seem to be helpful for such patients, but no systematic intervention studies have been performed. In adult patients, one also has to guard against unrealistic expectations from genital surgery, especially in patients who desire change from female to male. After careful consideration of the various pros and cons, some patients make a decision for a somewhat masculine ("butch") lesbian lifestyle rather than for a full transition to the male gender.

Individual case reports indicate that gender reassignments based on patients' wishes have been done at any age between early elementary school age and middle adulthood. The threshold for gender reassignment of gender-dysphoric children and adolescents with a somatic DSD is much lower than that for gender-dysphoric children without a somatic DSD.[10] The somatic DSD usually supplies a hormonal explanation for the gender change that at least seems plausible, even if it is not strictly demonstrable as a cause in an individual case. Genital surgery is common in infants and adolescents with a somatic DSD and is also done in middle childhood, especially when urinary function problems and urinary infections occur as a consequence of the DSD-caused configurations of the urogenital tract. Also, infertility is frequently already present in patients with a somatic DSD, unlike in gender-dysphoric patients without a somatic DSD, where the implication of likely later gonadectomy and attendant infertility tends to constitute an ethical and/or emotional barrier to gender reassignment on the part of many service providers.

Nevertheless, it seems prudent to make the decision on a social transition to the desired gender in patients with a somatic DSD only if there is a long-standing history of gender-atypical behavior and if gender dysphoria and/or the desire to change gender has been "strong and persistent," as formulated in DSM-IV-TR, for a considerable period such as at least 6 months, which is the period of full symptom expression required for the application of the gender dysphoria diagnosis as proposed for DSM-5 [the revision of DSM-IV's GID; see www.dsm5.org]. It helps the confidence with which the mental health provider makes the recommendation for gender reassignment if the direction of the desired gender change is in line with the long-term gender outcome reported in the scientific literature for the respective syndrome and degree of severity. A discrepancy here may increase caution and lead to a delay but should not be regarded as a definitive barrier to gender reassignment, provided the assessment has been thorough and the chronicity of the gender dysphoria has been well-established.

When the gender information is ambiguous or unclear or the patient's gender change wish is of rather recent origin, the original gender should be maintained and, especially, any gender-confirming genital surgery delayed. Under such circumstances the parents, of young children in particular, may need repeated explanations and support.

It is desirable that gender-dysphoric patients with a DSD undergo a prolonged period of living in the desired gender in most or all domains of everyday life as appropriate for the patient's age before undergoing any poorly reversible or irreversible medical treatment such as cross-gender hormone treatment or gender-confirming genital surgery. Such a real-life experience of 3 months has been recommended by the international standards of care for GIDs (without a DSD) as a requirement for cross-gender hormone treatment and of 2 years as a requirement for gender reassignment surgery.[38] In the absence of consensus-based guidelines for gender-dysphoric patients with a DSD and a solid empirical evidence base for such policies, the author tends to orient recommendations—cautiously and flexibly—using the eligibility and readiness criteria of these standards. Many patients who come to the author from remote parts of the United States or from foreign countries have already been living in the desired gender for years; in such cases one just has to obtain reliable confirmation from other family members and/or romantic partners that such an implicit real-life experience has actually taken place, and the patient's experience of this period needs to be evaluated in detail by the clinician.

SUMMARY

The gender-dysphoric patient with a DSD presents a challenge for the mental health services provider, because clinical assistance must be based on an understanding of the medical and psychosocial situation of the patient in his or her cultural context, with the implications for future gender development, sexual functioning, and related quality of life. Yet the empirical data base in this area of rare syndromes and rare mental health specialists is still very limited. Moreover, the care of non-DSD persons with gender dysphoria is currently undergoing rapid change, as shown in other articles in this issue. Although many of the psychologic/psychiatric assessment methods are applicable to both groups of patients, the DSD-specific aspects of presentation and medical context argue for caution and flexibility when applying guidelines developed for non-DSD gender-dysphoric patients to those with a DSD.

REFERENCES

1. Hughes IA, Houk C, Ahmed SF, et al. Consensus statement on management of intersex disorders. Arch Dis Child 2006;91:554–63.
2. Grumbach MM, Hughes IA, Conte FA. Disorders of sex differentiation. In: Larsen PR, Kronenberg HM, Mehmed S, Polonsky, KS editors. Williams textbook of endocrinology. 10th edition. Philadelphia: WB Saunders; 2003. p. 842–1002.
3. Meyer-Bahlburg HFL. Gender assignment in intersexuality. J Psychol Human Sex 1998;10:1–21.
4. Meyer-Bahlburg HFL. Gender dysphoria and gender change in persons with intersexuality: Introduction. Arch Sex Behav 2005;34:371–73.
5. Dessens AB, Slijper FME, Drop SLS. Gender dysphoria and gender change in chromosomal females with congenital adrenal hyperplasia. Arch Sex Behav 2005;34: 389–97.
6. Cohen-Kettenis PT. Gender change in 46,XY persons with 5?-reductase-2 deficiency and 17?-hydroxysteroid dehydrogenase-3 deficiency. Arch Sex Behav 2005;34:399–410.
7. Mazur T. Gender dysphoria and gender change in androgen insensitivity or micropenis. Arch Sex Behav 2005;34:411–21.
8. Meyer-Bahlburg HFL. Gender identity outcome in female-raised 46,XY persons with penile agenesis, cloacal exstrophy of the bladder, or penile ablation. Arch Sex Behav 2005;34:423–38.
9. Zucker KJ, Lawrence AA. Epidemiology of gender identity disorder: recommendations for the Standards of Care of the World Professional Association for Transgender Health. International Journal of Transgenderism 2009;11:8–18.
10. Meyer-Bahlburg HFL. Variants of gender differentiation in somatic disorders of sex development: recommendations for version 7 of the World Professional Association for Transgender Health's Standards of Care. International Journal of Transgenderism 2009; 11:226–37.

11. American Psychiatric Association. Diagnostic and statistical manual of mental disorders. 4th edition. Treatment revision. Washington, DC: American Psychiatric Publishing; 2000.

12. Meyer-Bahlburg HFL. Treatment guidelines for children with disorders of sex development. Neuropsychiatr Enfance Adolesc 2008;56:345–49.

13. Ruble DN, Martin CL, Berenbaum SA. Gender development. In: Damon W, Lerner RM, Eisenberg N, editors. Handbook of child psychology. Social, emotional, and personal development. Vol 3. 6th edition. New York: J. Wiley & Sons; 2006. p. 858–932.

14. Martin CL, Ruble DN. Patterns of gender development. Annu Rev Psychol 2009;61: 353–81.

15. Money J, Ehrhardt AA. Man and woman, boy and girl: the differentiation and dimorphism of gender identity from conception to maturity. Baltimore (MD): The Johns Hopkins University Press; 1972.

16. Speiser PW, Azziz R, Baskin LS, et al. Congenital adrenal hyperplasia due to steroid 21-hydroxylase deficiency. An Endocrine Society clinical practice guideline. J Clin Endocrinol Metab 2010;95:4133–60.

17. Warne GI, Bhatia V. Intersex, East and West. In: Sytsma S, editor. Ethics and intersex. Berlin: Springer; 2006. p. 183–205.

18. Uslu R, Oztop D, Ozcan O, et al. Factors contributing to sex assignment and reassignment decisions in Turkish children with 46,XY disorders of sex development. J Pediatr Endocrinol Metab 2007;20:1001–15.

19. Zucker KJ. Measurement of psychosexual differentiation. Arch Sex Behav 2005;34: 375–88.

20. Achenbach TM. Child Behavior Checklist for Ages 1 1/2–5. Burlington (VT): ASEBA, University of Vermont; 2000.

21. Golombok S, Rust J. The Pre-School Activities Inventory: a standardized assessment of gender role in children. Psychol Assess 1993;5:131–6.

22. Meyer-Bahlburg HFL, Dolezal C, Baker SW, et al. Prenatal androgenization affects gender-related behavior but not gender identity in 5–12 year old girls with congenital adrenal hyperplasia. Arch Sex Behav 2004;33:97–104.

23. Zucker KJ, Doering RW, Bradley SJ, et al. Sex-typed play in gender-disturbed children: a comparison to sibling and psychiatric controls. Arch Sex Behav 1982;11: 309–21.

24. Zucker KJ, Finegan JK, Doering RW, et al. Human figure drawings of gender-problem children: a comparison to sibling, psychiatric, and normal controls. J Abnorm Child Psychol 1983;11:287–98.

25. Zucker KJ, Bradley SJ, Lowry Sullivan CB, et al. A gender identity interview for children. J Pers Assess 1993;61:443–56.

26. Achenbach TM. Child Behavior Checklist for Ages 6–18. Burlington (VT): ASEBA, University of Vermont; 2001.

27. Meyer-Bahlburg HFL, Sandberg DE, Dolezal CL, et al. Gender-related assessment of childhood play. J Abnorm Child Psychol 1994;22:643–60.

28. Meyer-Bahlburg HFL, Sandberg DE, Yager TJ, et al. Questionnaire scales for the assessment of atypical gender development in girls and boys. J Psychol Human Sex 1994;6:19–39.

29. Johnson LL, Bradley SJ, Birkenfeld-Adams AS, et al. A parent-report Gender Identity Questionnaire for Children. Arch Sex Behav 2004;33:105–16.

30. Achenbach TM. Youth Self Report for Ages 11–18. Burlington (VT): ASEBA, University of Vermont; 2001.

31. Lippa R. Gender-related individual differences and psychological adjustment in terms of the Big Five and circumplex models. J Pers Soc Psychol 1995;61:1184–202.
32. Meyer-Bahlburg HFL, Dolezal C, Baker SW, et al. Gender development in women with congenital adrenal hyperplasia as a function of disorder severity. Arch Sex Behav 2006;35:667–84.
33. Berenbaum SA. Effects of early androgens on sex-typed activities and interests in adolescents with congenital adrenal hyperplasia. Horm Behav 1999;35:102–10.
34. Meyer-Bahlburg HFL, Dolezal C, Zucker KJ, et al. The Recalled Childhood Gender Questionnaire-Revised: a psychometric analysis in a sample of women with congenital adrenal hyperplasia. J Sex Res 2006;43:364–7.
35. Meyer-Bahlburg HFL, Dolezal C, Johnson LL, et al. Development and validation of the Pregnancy and Infant Orientation Questionnaire. J Sex Res 2010;47:598–610.
36. Deogracias JJ, Johnson LL, Meyer-Bahlburg HFL, et al. The Gender Identity/Gender Dysphoria Questionnaire for Adolescents and Adults. J Sex Res 2007;44:370–79.
37. Singh D, Deogracias JJ, Johnson LL, et al. The Gender Identity/Gender Dysphoria Questionnaire for Adolescents and Adults: further validity evidence. J Sex Res 2010;47:49–58.
38. Meyer W III, Bockting WO, Cohen-Kettenis P, et al. The Harry Benjamin International Gender Dysphoria Association's standards of care for gender identity disorders. 6th version. J Psychol Human Sex 2001;13:1–34.

Development of AACAP Practice Parameters for Gender Nonconformity and Gender Discordance in Children and Adolescents

Stewart L. Adelson, MD[a,b,*]

KEYWORDS

- Adolescent • Child • Gender identity • Practice guideline
- Gender nonconformity • Gender discordance

The American Academy of Child and Adolescent Psychiatry (AACAP) is preparing a publication, *Practice Parameter on Gay, Lesbian or Bisexual Sexual Orientation, Gender-Nonconformity, and Gender Discordance in Children and Adolescents*. This practice parameter is the first guideline of its kind produced by a leading psychiatric organization on the mental health needs of these groups of children and adolescents. The purpose of this article is to describe the process of development of the parameter and to provide background information about the rationale for its contents and organization, with an emphasis on the parameter's information about gender non-conformity and gender discordance in children and adolescents. This report includes information about key scientific and clinical issues, definitions of basic terms, and concepts of psychosexual development including links between sexual orientation and gender development in children and adolescents.

AACAP develops and publishes practice parameters on a wide variety of topics. These topics include practice parameters on clinical topics like depression, anxiety, and learning disorders; on other topics related to clinical practice such as school consultation or seclusion and restraint; and on special populations. AACAP practice parameters are intended to provide state-of-the-art clinical and scientific knowledge on a wide variety of topics to help guide the field of child and adolescent psychiatry and related professions. There are two basic kinds of AACAP practice parameters:

[a] Division of Child and Adolescent Psychiatry, Columbia University College of Physicians and Surgeons, New York, NY, USA
[b] Division of Child and Adolescent Psychiatry, Weil Medical College of Cornell University, New York, NY, USA
* Corresponding author. 117 West 17th Street, Suite 2B, New York, NY 10011.
E-mail address: sla15@columbia.edu

Child Adolesc Psychiatric Clin N Am 20 (2011) 651–663
doi:10.1016/j.chc.2011.07.001
childpsych.theclinics.com
1056-4993/11/$ – see front matter © 2011 Elsevier Inc. All rights reserved.

patient-oriented and clinician-oriented. Patient-oriented parameters are intended to provide best treatment practices based on empirical evidence and clinical consensus; examples include topics such as bipolar disorder and schizophrenia. Clinician-oriented parameters are intended to provide caregivers with practice principles to foster clinical skills. The *Practice Parameter on Gay, Lesbian or Bisexual Sexual Orientation, Gender-Nonconformity, and Gender Discordance in Children and Adolescents* is a clinician-oriented parameter related to these special populations. At the heart of the practice parameters lies a list of clinical principles to guide clinicians on key concepts related to practice. The topics addressed by the principles in clinician-oriented parameters are based upon expert opinion derived from clinical experience. These principles are elaborated upon in the text of the parameter, which includes empirical evidence that forms the foundation of the clinical principles.

The development of AACAP practice parameters is overseen by the AACAP Committee on Quality Issues (CQI; formerly the Work Group on Quality Issues [WGQI]). A consensus committee convened by the CQI and the AACAP Council review and approve final practice parameters before they are published and released to the general public. In October 2005, members of AACAP's Sexual Orientation and Gender Identity Issues Committee (SOGIIC) met in Toronto during AACAP's annual meeting to discuss a request from AACAP's WGQI to develop practice parameters on children and adolescents who were growing up as members of sexual minorities. They met as a committee and with the WGQI/CQI several times a year in formal meetings to discuss the parameters. Development of the parameter has been the result of a collaborative process over approximately 6 years among the CQI and members of the SOGIIC committee, as well as several members of the Lesbian and Gay Child and Adolescent Psychiatric Association (LAGCAPA). The author is a member of SOGIIC.

Early in the process, SOGIIC and members of LAGCAPA, under guidance from CQI, decided to use as the main portion in an early draft of the parameter a text and bibliography that the author had previously researched and written for a class on gay and lesbian youth in the combined Columbia/Cornell child and adolescent psychiatry residency program. Subsequently, members of SOGIIC and LAGCAPA assigned this author the role of primary author of the practice parameter. The author researched and wrote most of the remaining text, including the introduction, background material on gender nonconformity and gender discordance, and most of the text of the practice principles that had been drafted by the group in their initial meetings. In addition, the author edited and incorporated into a coherent whole sections of briefer preliminary writings drafted by several SOGIIC members in subsequent revisions. During this process of the practice parameter's development, SOGIIC and members of LAGCAPA met approximately biannually in person and by conference call and communicated regularly between formal meetings to oversee, review, comment on, and approve successive drafts. In addition, several topic experts assisted the SOGIIC committee by reviewing the document and making suggestions. The members of the CQI, SOGIIC, and the topic experts are to be listed in the practice parameter. The AACAP general membership also provided feedback including comments, questions, and suggestions about the draft document on the AACAP Web site from September 2010 through January 2011 and also at an open member forum at the AACAP annual meeting in New York on October 28, 2010.

From the outset, a key objective of CQI and SOGIIC was to produce a practice parameter that would be supported by objective evidence, that reflects expert consensus, and that is transparent about areas of controversy or where consensus is lacking. To achieve this, CQI and SOGIIC established a method for preparing the parameter that is intended to be both free from bias and also transparent about any possible conflict of interest. In order to avoid bias, clinical principles had to be supported by evidence in the scientific literature assembled through a search and winnowed in a transparent process using an explicit, objective strategy. The clinical principles and text of the parameter were continually reviewed, refined, and updated under guidance from CQI to assure that they were supported by evidence. In addition to freedom from bias, to assure transparency about any possible conflict of interest, authors and expert reviewers were required to disclose any conflicts on the AACAP Web site during the period of membership review of the draft parameter and also in the published parameter.

The details of the process of preparing and assembling references for the parameter are discussed in its Methodology section. Briefly, the references were obtained by online searches of Medline and PsycINFO databases. A search of relevant PsychINFO and Medline keyword terms produced 7825 references. A subsequent search of relevant PsychINFO thesaurus terms (descriptors) produced 1847 references, and of relevant Medline MeSH (medical subject headings) produced 2855 references. The specific search terms and parameters used in the search are described in the practice parameter's Methodology section. In addition, searches of relevant publications by experts and related articles, bibliographies of source materials including books,[1-3] book chapters,[4] and review articles[5-7] yielded further references. These experts are also identified in the practice parameter's Methodology section. Discussions at scientific meetings in the past decade were also considered.

Only references based on literature review, published in peer-reviewed literature, or based on methodologically sound strategies such as use of population-based, controlled, blinded, prospective, or multisite evidence were used. A set was selected whose primary focus was mental health related to sexual orientation, gender nonconformity, and gender discordance in children and adolescents and that illustrated key points related to clinical practice. Preference was given to references that were more recent, relevant to the US population, most illustrative of key clinical concepts, or based upon larger samples, prospective study design, or metaanalysis. A representative sample of references presenting different viewpoints was selected when discussing issues around which consensus is not yet established in the field.

TERMINOLOGY AND DEFINITIONS

The practice parameter includes a section on definitions of terms related to sexual orientation and gender development. One challenge in writing the practice parameter resulted from the fact that many terms related to sexual development are being continually updated. As concepts evolve, terms are in flux and the semantic boundaries between them shift. For example, the term *gender role behavior* is used in some contexts in a "social constructionist" sense, with the perspective that gender-related phenomena and their meaning are contingent upon social factors such as language and culture (for example, to refer to social phenomena such as whether women or men do housework or have professional careers). However, as knowledge has grown about biological influences on certain gender role behaviors, the meaning of the term *gender role behavior* has been used in other contexts in a different, "essentialist" sense, with a perspective that some gender-related phenomena such as childhood patterns of rough-and-tumble play, levels of motoric activity, and degrees of physical aggression are influenced by biological factors operating independently from of social context or influence. In the practice parameters, an effort was made to define the term *gender role behavior* in a way that acknowledges both perspectives and the possibility of both biological and social determinants.

When contentious issues regarding gender are debated in the literature from opposing theoretical vantage points, language and terminology can acquire connotations of affiliation with one intellectual camp or another. In recent years, the term *disorder of sexual differentiation* has been generally replaced by the term *disorder of sex development*. The former term may be construed as implying the empirical truth of a binary conceptualization of gender, which some may question; the latter term is more neutral in this regard, although it allows for the possibility of binary phenomena such as the biological polarity of genital and brain anlage. In keeping with the development in the literature, the practice parameter uses the latter, current term.

In addition, certain terms may acquire an anachronistic patina over time. For example, the terms *gender atypical* and *gender variant* may imply strangeness or abnormality with vague connotations of judgmentalism to some. These terms seem to be used less commonly in the recent scientific literature than the term *gender nonconforming*. The practice parameter includes all three terms in the definitions in order to familiarize readers with terms in the scientific literature, but uses the more current one, *gender nonconforming,* in its title and text. Finally, some terms may seem to presuppose concepts of pathology that are debated; for example, the *Diagnostic and Statistical Manual of Mental Disorders,* 4th edition (DSM-IV) diagnosis of gender identity disorder (GID)[8,9] has been controversial, in part because it uses pathological terminology for a condition whose status as a disorder is debated in the scientific literature. A particular effort was made to use terminology that does not presuppose any outcome of current debates over issues such as the status of GID as a diagnosis, but rather that anticipates a range of possible outcomes as much as possible and strives to use terms that, as far as one can tell, make the document useful for as long as possible.

Ultimately, science and society must be able to meet in a forum in which they can converse about gender. In order to have a meaningful discussion, the terminology used must be scientifically and medically precise, neither dogmatic nor parochial, and suitable to convey coherent thoughts in the conversations of all parties who meet and participate in the discussion. Ideally, using suitable terminology, science can address objective questions that are asked within a cultural context. In writing the practice parameters, an effort was made to define terms in a way that reflects current usage and is neutral regarding any intellectual perspective or agenda. The terms were gleaned from the literature, and their definitions vetted with experts and subjected to peer review. Given the ever-evolving nature of language, terminology will unquestionably change in the future. Such change is a reflection of the living nature of ideas and language, and is as it should be. The terms in the practice parameter may have a limited shelf life, but with any luck the expiration date will not be too soon.

OVERALL SCOPE AND BASIC ORGANIZATION

The *Practice Parameter on Gay, Lesbian or Bisexual Sexual Orientation, Gender-Nonconformity, and Gender Discordance in Children and Adolescents* includes discussion of diverse populations and issues. For example, homosexuality, which was eliminated as a DSM (ie, American Psychiatric Association) diagnosis in 1973, is quite different from GID, which remains a DSM diagnosis (albeit a controversial one).[9] At the inception of the project, members of SOGIIC considered whether to develop two separate parameters—one dealing with matters of sexual orientation and the other with matters of gender development—or one comprehensive parameter that dealt with both issues.

Although sexual orientation and gender development are distinct topics that might have been considered in separate parameters, SOGIIC decided in an early meeting that a comprehensive parameter dealing with both topics was preferable. It reached this conclusion because review of the literature showed clinically significant relationships between lines of development in gender and sexual orientation. In addition, there are important clinical distinctions to be made among a variety of issues in gender development affecting children and adolescents, such as the difference between gender identity, gender nonconformity, and gender discordance and the unique relation of each of these to the issue of sexual orientation. The committee believed that a single comprehensive parameter could best discuss, compare, and contrast these issues in a way that would avoid unnecessary confusion and produce a useful document for working clinicians and other mental health professionals.

The parameter is divided into separate topics, including a section on homosexuality and another on gender identity and gender discordance. A subsection on psychosexual development and homosexual orientation (contained within the section on homosexuality) describes various developmental trajectories of sexual orientation and gender-related issues. Information is included about influences on development, including biological and social influences on homosexuality, gender nonconformity, and gender discordance, and on important clinical issues related to these in children and adolescents. The general content of the parameter and the rationale for decisions about what is included are described later.

GENDER DEVELOPMENT

The practice parameter reviews information from the scientific literature on various lines of gender development. This review includes information about the development of both gender identity and gender role behaviors, and also the developmental lines along which these are organized. In the parameter, gender identity is defined as an individual's personal sense of self as male or female. The literature indicates that gender identity usually is established by approximately 3 years of age, is concordant with sex (which refers to anatomical sex) and gender (which refers to the perception of one's sex as male or female), and is stable over the lifetime.

The practice parameter defines gender role behavior as activities, interests, and use of symbols, styles, or other personal and social attributes that are recognized as masculine or feminine[10,11] and are distinct from sex, gender, gender identity, or erotic feelings and fantasies. Gender role behaviors involve gender differences in areas such as patterns of play, interpersonal behavior, and use of styles and symbols. The parameter discusses patterns of gender role behavior that generally differ between boys and girls. These differences include patterns of motoric activity, predilection for rough-and-tumble play, patterns in displaying aggression physically as opposed to socially, toy selection in experimental protocols using unstructured play opportunities with a choice among a range of toys, and the use of styles and symbols that are recognized in society as being masculine or feminine in gesture, speech, grooming, and dress. The practice parameter describes evidence that there is an interactive influence among social, psychological, and biological factors on childhood gender role behavior and gender identity.[12–14]

GENDER NONCONFORMITY

The practice parameter defines childhood gender nonconformity as variation from norms in gender role behavior such as toy preferences, rough-and-tumble play, aggression, or playmate gender (equivalent to the terms *gender variance* and *gender atypicality*) and discusses the fact that some children display sex-atypical patterns of gender-related behaviors.[13] It provides examples of gender nonconformity such as aversion to rough-and-tumble play and vigorous tomboyishness among girls.

The practice parameter includes a section on biological factors that seem to influence both gender nonconformity in childhood and sexual orientation in adulthood.[15] This section includes evidence of a possible effect of prenatal sex hormones on gender role behavior in childhood and sexual orientation in adulthood.[16,17] It also includes discussion of evidence that certain neuroanatomical features may correlate with sexual orientation.[15,18] The parameter discusses limitations on the conclusions that can be drawn from these findings and the need for further research to establish their significance.

GENDER NONCONFORMITY AND HOMOSEXUALITY

The practice parameter includes information about the developmental relationship between childhood gender nonconformity and adult homosexuality in both males[19] and females (in whom childhood gender nonconformity is sometimes associated with adult homosexual orientation, although less consistently than in males).[20] Information is presented based upon retrospective data from studies conducted in several diverse cultures suggesting that this association is a fairly common pattern and may be one normal developmental pathway toward adult homosexuality, especially in males.[21,22]

SOGIIC decided to include this information on the developmental association between childhood gender nonconformity and adult homosexuality in part because it is a clinically important one, as it seems to account for the report of many gay and lesbian people that they felt "different" from others in childhood for reasons other than erotic orientation. It may be associated with clinically important phenomena, such as low peer status and poor self-esteem (especially in boys)[23] and peer harassment, which can have important long-term mental health consequences. These clinical phenomena are addressed in the parameter's practice principles. The parameter discusses information about the association of these phenomena with significant distress, psychological symptoms, family problems stemming from a poor developmental fit between children's gender-nonconformity or sexual orientation and parents' expectations, and social problems.[4,24]

The practice parameter includes discussion of clinical issues in sexual minority youth that are related to the social and psychological consequences of gender nonconformity in children and adolescents. These issues include sexual prejudice (also known as heterosexism, or, more commonly, homophobia), which is defined in the parameter as bias against homosexual people. Although the term *homophobia* is a prejudice rather than a phobia and thus technically a misnomer, since the term is nevertheless frequently used colloquially, SOGIIC decided to include it alongside the semantically more logical term *sexual prejudice* in the definitions and to use it in the text of the parameter in order to realistically reflect the way youth and families speak.[25] Related to sexual prejudice and homophobia, the parameter also highlights the phenomenon of internalized sexual prejudice or internalized homophobia, which it defines as a syndrome of self-loathing based upon the adoption of antihomosexual attitudes, beliefs, and values of the aggressor by homosexual people themselves. The parameter discusses a variety of stressors and psychological mechanisms that can trigger this phenomenon.[1,6]

The practice parameter also includes information about the clinical importance for homosexual youth of the unique developmental experience of coping with sexual feelings that are discrepant from family and societal expectations. It discusses conflicts over revealing a homosexual identity to others (coming out).[26] This discussion highlights the effect of a developmental history of gender nonconformity in childhood on adolescents' development of gender-based self-esteem and ability to cope with this conflict. It discusses the risk for chronic anxiety and depression as well as the difficulty of establishing identity and independence adaptively in adolescence.

The practice parameter includes information on risks such as suicide in gay and lesbian adolescents.[27–29] Included is information on the possible association of a history of prominent childhood gender nonconformity with risk for suicidality in gay adolescents.[30] Homosexuality, especially when associated with childhood gender nonconformity, may be a relative risk factor for other problems such as mood disorder, anxiety, substance abuse, or suicidality. These comorbidities may be mediated by social intolerance. Also discussed is evidence that the developmental interval between first same-sex sexual experience and self-labeling as gay may be a period of particular risk for suicide in gay teens.[29]

Also included is information on high-risk sexual behavior and substance abuse. The practice parameter discusses how the effects of gender nonconformity on the development of self-esteem and consolidation of identity may mediate risk behaviors.

GENDER DISCORDANCE

In addition to information on gender nonconformity, the practice parameter includes information on gender discordance in children and adolescents. Gender discordance is defined in the parameter as a discrepancy between anatomical sex and gender identity. Related terms are also defined, including the term *gender identity variance*, which refers to a spectrum of gender-discordant phenomena; *transgender* youth, defined as youth who have a gender identity that is discordant from their anatomical sex; and *transsexual* youth, defined as transgender youth who make their perceived gender and/or anatomical sex conform with their gender identity through strategies such as dress, grooming, hormone use and/or surgery (a process defined as *sex reassignment* or *gender reassignment*).

The practice parameter discusses controversies in the diagnosis of GID. In keeping with the AACAP mandate governing areas of controversy in practice parameters, a representative range of various viewpoints about issues is presented to reflect the current state of the field, with no assumption about the ultimate resolution of controversy. The parameter includes information on controversies such as whether the diagnosis represents a medicalization of a social prejudice, whether the distress and dysfunction that are associated with gender discordance and a criterion of GID are the result of that prejudice, and whether GID represents an iatrogenic condition resulting from medical accommodation of a body dysmorphia that is inconsistent with the medical response to other nongender-related body dysmorphias. Also discussed are controversies about whether young children are always able or willing to verbalize cross-gender wishes, which is in turn related to a debate about whether a verbalized wish to be the opposite gender should remain a criterion of GID in children.

At the time of writing of the AACAP practice parameter, the American Psychiatric Association (APA) was simultaneously reviewing the diagnosis of GID in anticipation of the publication of DSM-5 (R.R. Pleak, personal communication, 2011). An effort was made to write the AACAP practice parameter in a way that presupposes no particular outcome of APA process regarding the status of GID as a diagnosis or its criteria, in the hope that the AACAP practice parameter remains a useful document following its completion and the publication of DSM-5 by the APA (see www.dsm5.org and the article in this issue by Zucker).

DEVELOPMENTAL TRAJECTORIES OF GENDER DISCORDANCE

The practice parameter discusses different categories of gender discordance emerging in childhood, adolescence, or adulthood, which may be influenced by different factors and which are characterized by unique developmental trajectories that largely determine whether gender discordance is persistent or transient.[31] Data are presented that when gender discordance presents before puberty it persists into adulthood only 2.2%[32] to 11.9%[33] of the time; in contrast, gender discordance presenting in adolescence usually persists through adulthood,[34] often leading to adult transsexualism.

The practice parameter discusses the developmental relationship between gender discordance in childhood and later homosexuality. The different developmental trajectories of gender discordance also differ in whether there is a posttransition homosexual or heterosexual orientation. As gender discordance fades, 75% of boys with GID become homosexual or bisexual in fantasy and 80% in behavior by age 19.[33] Therefore, like gender nonconformity, gender discordance is developmentally related to homosexuality. However, it appears to constitute a distinct set of developmental lines, which are described in the parameter.

The practice parameter includes information on a number of biological, neuroanatomic, neuropsychological and neurophysiologic markers that have been described in association with gender discordance but not gender nonconformity or homosexuality,[35,36] as well as evidence of the influence of prenatal sex hormones on gender identity.[37] It also discusses several hypothesized social influences on gender discordance. A review of the literature yielded no controlled empirical evidence in support of these hypothesis to date.[32,38,39]

CLINICAL ISSUES IN GENDER DISCORDANCE

The practice parameter discusses clinically important information on comorbid psychopathology in children and adolescents with gender discordance including behavior problems and anxiety.[40,41] Controversies regarding the cause of this comorbid psychopathology are also discussed, including questions about whether it is the result of family and social rejection, of psychological distress due to the real discrepancy between psychological and anatomic gender, or whether it is due to maternal and family psychopathology, which is hypothesized to also cause gender discordance.[34,39] A search of the literature also found no controlled scientific studies to test these various hypotheses.

The practice parameter contains a section pertaining to the treatment of GID. Review of the literature reveals that there is debate not only about the diagnosis of GID and its criteria in children but also on treatment approaches for GID and gender discordance and, to some degree, what the goals of treatment should be. At the time of this writing, the APA has a task force on gender identity disorder that is addressing the need for treatment guidelines to be developed by the APA (R/R. Pleak, personal communication, 2011). The parameter includes discussion of early treatment approaches for GID and gender discordance from the 1970s based on behavioral paradigms[42] as well as ethical concerns that these approaches are inappropriately punitive and coercive[43] and the lack of long-term follow-up in controlled studies of their potential benefits and harms. The parameter also describes other treatment approaches advocated for GID, including psychodynamic psychotherapy.[38]

The parameter discusses recently proposed goals of treatment for gender discordance arising in childhood, which include reducing gender discordance, decreasing social ostracism, and reducing psychiatric comorbidity.[7] It describes a variety of treatment approaches that embrace these goals to varying degrees, especially in regard to whether hastening the desistence (ie, fading) of gender discordance is an explicit goal of treatment. In order to illustrate a range of opinion on this matter, the practice parameter describes two treatment strategies based on uncontrolled case series focusing on parent guidance and peer group interaction. One seeks to hasten desistence of gender discordance in boys through eclectic relationship-focused and milieu-focused interventions;[44] another encourages tolerance of gender discordance while setting limits on expression of gender-discordant behavior to the extent that these limits are necessary to decrease risk for peer or community harassment.[45] Even though the degree varies to which desistence of gender discordance is a goal of these contrasting approaches, desistence has nevertheless been described in both treatment approaches, as it is in untreated children.

In addition to the proposed benefits of treatment, the parameter discusses several possible risks of treatment. These include the risk that children will learn to simply hide their gender-discordant wishes in response to treatment, that they may be traumatized by disapproval of their gender discordance, and that treatment may incur family rejection of gender-discordant children. These risks are discussed in light of the fact that family rejection is associated with problems such as depression, suicidality, and substance abuse in gay youth.[24]

In preparing the practice parameter, no evidence was found of any randomized, controlled trials of the efficacy of any treatment aimed at eliminating gender discordance. As a result of the potential risks of treatment and evidence that gender discordance persists in only a small minority of untreated cases arising in childhood, the parameter concludes that no treatment to eliminate gender discordance can be endorsed at this time. It calls for further research on predictors of persistence and desistence of childhood gender discordance and outlines open ethical questions on the long-term risks and benefits of intervention that must be addressed before any treatment to eliminate gender discordance can be endorsed.

The parameter highlights unique clinical features of the developmental trajectory of gender discordance presenting in adolescence or adulthood[46] and how these differ from clinical issues of gender discordance in childhood. Included in this developmental trajectory is the distress that gender-discordant adolescents can feel in puberty when secondary sex characteristics emerge. Because gender discordance presenting in adolescence or adulthood seems much more likely to persist than that presenting in childhood, the practice parameter describes treatment approaches for adolescents that assume persistence of gender discordance. These treatment approaches focus on management of comorbid psychiatric issues such as depression, anxiety, and anger in addition to general behavioral and emotional problems and functioning and also on management of risks to transsexuals of sex reassignment efforts that are not medically managed, such as the use of illicitly obtained sex hormones or other medications with hormonal activity in an effort to bring biological sex into conformity with gender identity.

The parameter includes evidence from recent research on novel treatments for adolescents involving sex hormone suppression under endocrinologic management with psychiatric consultation when decisions about sex reassignment cannot be deferred until adulthood. In such treatment, gonadotropin-releasing hormone analogues are used to reversibly delay development of secondary sexual characteristics.[46] The parameter discusses use of such treatment to avoid distress about secondary sexual characteristics, minimize the later need for surgery to reverse them, and delay the need for treatment decisions until maturity allows informed consent.[7]

The parameter describes evidence on the benefits and tolerability of such treatment[47] and possible benefit in preventing later adult mental health problems.[48]

COMPARISON OF GENDER NONCONFORMITY AND GENDER DISCORDANCE

The practice parameter compares and contrasts the phenomenology of gender discordance and gender nonconformity. It points out that children and adolescents may be gender-nonconforming while displaying a gender identity that is concordant with their anatomic sex. It discusses gender discordance as a core feature of GID as defined in DSM-IV.[9] Gender nonconformity in and of itself does not meet criteria for GID or any other DSM diagnosis. Information is presented that the prevalence of gender discordance may be quite low but that there are challenges in measuring it.

Gender-discordant children may also be gender-nonconforming; both traits are required for the diagnosis of GID according to DSM-IV criteria. However, several differences distinguish gender nonconformity from gender discordance. Many children with gender nonconformity do not display gender discordance and may in fact be extremely distressed by feelings of being perceived as insufficiently masculine (in the case of boys) or feminine (in the case of girls). Furthermore, gender-nonconforming children are characterized by different developmental trajectories: gender nonconformity emerges in childhood, whereas gender discordance can emerge in childhood, adolescence, or adulthood. Additionally, the biological markers discussed previously that are associated with gender nonconformity and gender discordance differ.

Although gender nonconformity and gender discordance differ in their clinical features, developmental trajectories, and biological markers and therefore seem to be discrete phenomena, the practice parameter includes information on factors that may affect the ability to distinguish these phenomena in research and clinical settings. These factors include the possibility that shame will cause children to be covert about gender nonconforming and discordant feelings and behaviors and the possible influence of family and social factors on the expression and perception of gender nonconforming and discordant feelings and behaviors. Related to these difficulties, the issue has been debated whether a verbal report of cross-gender wishes should be a criterion of GID in DSM-5. However, the fact that there may be difficulty distinguishing gender nonconformity from gender discordance does not mean these phenomena are the same. On the contrary, the difference seems to be both clinically significant and important to youth.

SUMMARY

The practice parameter that the AACAP is preparing on gay, lesbian, and bisexual sexual orientation, gender nonconformity, and gender discordance in children and adolescents subsumes clinically important topics related to both gender development and development of sexual orientation. Ethical issues in practice and research, areas of both consensus and controversy, and matters requiring further research are discussed in the parameter.

The scope and organization of the parameter reflects the multiple, distinct developmental lines related to gender identity, gender role behavior, gender nonconformity, and gender discordance. These developmental lines seem to be discrete, albeit sometimes related, phenomena with distinct developmental trajectories, biological correlations, and associated psychosexual and clinical phenomena. There are significant developmental relationships among these developmental lines and sexual orientation. The parameter includes information on the relationship of these developmental phenomena to one another and to important clinical issues in children and adolescents. These issues include the development of self-esteem and risk for outcomes such as depression, anxiety, suicidal thought and behavior, substance abuse, and high-risk behavior. The practice parameter provides clinician-oriented practice principles based on current knowledge and evidence assembled by a method established by AACAP to guard against bias and conflict of interest.

ACKNOWLEDGMENTS

The author wishes to thank Joan Kinlan, MD, and Christopher Bellonci, MD, who made significant contributions to the practice parameter by serving as liaisons between the American Academy of Child and Adolescent Psychiatry's Committee on Quality Issues (CQI), Sexual Orientation and Gender Identity Issues Committee (SOGIIC), and Lesbian and Gay Child and Adolescent Psychiatry Association (LAGCAPA), as well as the members of CQI, SOGIIC, and LAGCAPA for their contributions to the practice parameter.

REFERENCES

1. Drescher J. Psychoanalytic therapy and the gay man. Hillsdale (NJ): Analytic Press; 1998.
2. Friedman RC. Male homosexuality: a contemporary psychoanalytic perspective. New Haven (CT): Yale University Press; 1988.
3. Friedman RC, Downey JI. Sexual orientation and psychoanalysis: sexual science and clinical practice. New York: Columbia University Press; 2002.
4. Friedman RC. The issue of homosexuality in psychoanalysis. In: Fonagy P, Krause R, Leuzinger-Bohleber M, Leuzinger-Bohleber M, eds. Identity, gender, and sexuality: 150 years after Freud. London: International Psychoanalytical Association; 2006. p. 79–102.
5. Friedman RC, Downey JI. Homosexuality. N Engl J Med 1994;331(14):923–30.
6. Savin-Williams RC, Cohen KM. Homoerotic development during childhood and adolescence. Child Adolesc Psychiatr Clin N Am 2004;13(3):529–49, vii.
7. Zucker KJ. Gender identity development and issues. Child Adolesc Psychiatr Clin N Am 2004;13(3):551–68, vii.
8. American Psychiatric Association. Diagnostic and statistical manual of mental disorders. 4th edition. Arlington (VA): American Psychiatric Publishing; 1994.
9. American Psychiatric Association. Diagnostic and statistical manual of mental disorders. 4th edition. Treatment revision. Arlington (VA): American Psychiatric Publishing; 2000.
10. Golombok S, Fivush R. Gender development. New York: Cambridge University Press; 1994.
11. Maccoby EE. The two sexes: growing up apart, coming together. The family and public policy. Cambridge (MA): Belknap Press of Harvard University Press; 1998.
12. Iervolino AC, Hines M, Golombok SE, et al. Genetic and environmental influences on sex-typed behavior during the preschool years. Child Dev 2005;76(4):826–40.
13. Ruble DN, Martin CL, Berenbaum SA. Gender development. In: Damon W, Lerner RM, editors. Handbook of child psychology. 6th edition [electronic resource]. Hoboken (NJ): Wiley InterScience; 2007. p. 858–932.
14. Bussey K, Bandura A. Social cognitive theory of gender development and differentiation. Psychol Rev 1999;106(4):676–713.
15. Mustanski BS, Chivers ML, Bailey JM. A critical review of recent biological research on human sexual orientation. Annu Rev Sex Res 2002;13:89–140.

16. Ellis L, Ames MA. Neurohormonal functioning and sexual orientation: a theory of homosexuality/heterosexuality. Psychol Bull 1987;101:233–58.
17. Meyer-Bahlburg HFL. Psychoendocrine research on sexual orientation: Current status and future options. Prog Brain Res 1984;61:375–98.
18. LeVay S. A difference in hypothalamic structure between heterosexual and homosexual men. Science 1991;253(5023):1034–7.
19. Whitam FL. The prehomosexual male child in three societies: the United States, Guatemala, Brazil. Arch Sex Behav 1980;9(2):87–99.
20. Whitam FL, Mathy RM. Childhood cross-gender behavior of homosexual females in Brazil, Peru, the Philippines, and the United States. Arch Sex Behav 1991;20(2):151–70.
21. Bell AP, Weinberg MS, Hammersmith SK. Sexual preference: its development in men and women. Bloomington (IN): Indiana University Press; 1981.
22. Bailey JM, Miller JS, Willerman L. Maternally rated childhood gender nonconformity in homosexuals and heterosexuals. Arch Sex Behav 1993;22:461–9.
23. Friedman RC, Downey JI. The psychobiology of late childhood: significance for psychoanalytic developmental theory and clinical practice. J Am Acad Psychoanal 2000;28(3):431–48.
24. Ryan C, Huebner D, Diaz RM, et al. Family rejection as a predictor of negative health outcomes in white and Latino lesbian, gay, and bisexual young adults. Pediatrics 2009;123(1):346–52.
25. Herdt G, van de Meer T. Homophobia and anti-gay violence— contemporary perspectives [editorial introduction]. Culture, Health & Sexuality 2003;5(2):99–101.
26. Carragher DJ, Rivers I. Trying to hide: a cross-national study of growing up for non-identified gay and bisexual male youth. Clin Child Psychol Psychiatry 2002;7:457–74.
27. Faulkner AH, Cranston K. Correlates of same-sex sexual behavior in a random sample of Massachusetts high school students. Am J Public Health 1998;88(2):262–6.
28. Garofalo R, Wolf RC, Kessel S, et al. The association between health risk behaviors and sexual orientation among a school-based sample of adolescents. Pediatrics 1998;101(5):895–902.
29. Remafedi G, French S, Story M, et al. The relationship between suicide risk and sexual orientation: results of a population-based study. Am J Public Health 1998;88(1):57–60.
30. Harry J. Parasuicide, gender, and gender deviance. J Health Soc Behav 1983;24(4):350–61.
31. Cohen-Kettenis PT, Gooren LJG. Transexualism: a review of etiology, diagnosis and treatment. J Psychosom Res 1999;46 (4):315–33.
32. Green R. The "sissy-boy syndrome" and the development of homosexuality. New Haven (CT): Yale University Press; 1987.
33. Zucker KJ, Bradley SJ. Gender identity disorder and psychosexual problems in children and adolescents. New York: Guilford; 1995.
34. Smith YL, van Goozen SH, Cohen-Kettenis PT. Adolescents with gender identity disorder who were accepted or rejected for sex reassignment surgery: a prospective follow-up study. J Am Acad Child Adolesc Psychiatry 2001;40(4):472–81.
35. Bradley SJ, Zucker KJ. Gender identity disorder: a review of the past 10 years. J Am Acad Child Adolesc Psychiatry 1997;36(7):872–80.
36. Zhou JN, Hofman MA, Gooren LJG, et al. A sex difference in the human brain and its relation to transexuality. Nature 1995;378:68–70.

37. Meyer-Bahlburg HF. Gender identity outcome in female-raised 46,XY persons with penile agenesis, cloacal exstrophy of the bladder, or penile ablation. Arch Sex Behav 2005;34(4):423–38.
38. Coates S, Friedman RC, Wolfe S. The etiology of boyhood gender identity disorder: A model for integrating temperament, development, and psychodynamics. Psychoanalytic Dialogues 1991;1(4):481–523.
39. Marantz S, Coates S. Mothers of boys with gender identity disorder: a comparison of matched controls. J Am Acad Child Adolesc Psychiatry 1991;30:310–5.
40. Cohen-Kettenis PT, Owen A, Kaijser VG, et al. Demographic characteristics, social competence, and behavior problems in children with gender identity disorder: a cross-national, cross-clinic comparative analysis. J Abnorm Child Psychol 2003; 31(1):41–53.
41. Zucker KJ, Owen A, Bradley SJ, et al. Gender-dysphoric children and adolescents: a comparative analysis of demographic characteristics and behavioral problems. Clin Child Psychol Psychiatry 2002;7:398–411.
42. Rekers GA, Kilgus M, Rosen AC. Long-term effects of treatment for gender identity disorder of childhood. J Psychol Human Sex 1990;3:121.
43. Pleak, RR. Ethical issues in diagnosing and treating gender-dysphoric children and adolescents. In: Rottnek M, editor. Sissies and tomboys: gender nonconformity and homosexual childhood. New York: New York University Press: 1999. p. 34–51.
44. Meyer-Bahlburg HFL. Gender identity disorder in young boys: a parent- and peer-based treatment protocol. Clin Child Psychol Psychiatry 2002;7:360–76.
45. Menvielle EJ, Tuerk C. A support group for parents of gender-nonconforming boys. J Am Acad Child Adolesc Psychiatry 2002;41(8):1010–3.
46. Hembree WC, Cohen-Kettenis P, Delemarre-van de Waal HA, et al. Endocrine treatment of transsexual persons: an endocrine society clinical practice guideline. J Clin Endocrinol Metab 2009;94(9):3132–54.
47. de Vries AL, Steensma TD, Doreleijers TA, et al. Puberty suppression in adolescents with gender identity disorder: a prospective follow-up study. J Sex Med 2010. [Epub ahead of print].
48. de Vries AL, Kreukels BP, Steensma TD, et al. Comparing adult and adolescent transsexuals: an MMPI-2 and MMPI-A study. Psychiatry Res 2010. [Epub ahead of print].

Assessment of Gender Variance in Children

Kenneth J. Zucker, PhD[a,b,*,†], Hayley Wood, PhD[a]

KEYWORDS

- Gender identity • Gender role • Gender variance
- Gender identity disorder • Assessment

This chapter will focus on the assessment of children who display gender-atypical behavior and, perhaps, identity. The aim is to provide an overview of assessment techniques that can be used clinically with children who show this behavioral pattern and that complement the routine use of DSM-IV[1] criteria for the diagnosis of gender identity disorder (GID) in clinical practice. It will also provide an overview of some common approaches to the assessment of other types of behavioral and socioemotional issues that may require clinical attention in these youngsters.

TERMINOLOGY

As a point of departure, it is important to delineate terminologic matters. There are an array of terms that can be used to characterize gender-related behavior in children. For example, the normative literature on gender development often uses the term "sex-typed behavior" (or "gender-typed behavior") to denote behaviors that, on average, distinguish the behaviors of boys and girls and that are consistent with cultural definitions of masculinity and femininity.[2] Some common examples of such behavior include peer affiliation preference, toy and activity interests, roles in fantasy/pretend play, and choice of apparel during dress-up play. Other examples are the propensity for engagement in rough-and-tumble play and parental rehearsal play. There are dozens, if not hundreds, of studies that have documented mean normative sex differences in these kinds of behaviors.[3] Other terms that one might encounter in the developmental literature include "sex-typical" versus "sex-atypical behavior" or "gender conformity" versus "gender nonconformity."

In the clinical setting, the diagnosis of GID is, in some respects, the gold standard in evaluation.[1] The diagnosis of GID is based on an appraisal of an array of sex-typed

Disclosure: The authors have nothing to disclose.
[a] Gender Identity Service, Child, Youth, and Family Program, Centre for Addiction and Mental Health, 250 College Street, Toronto, ON M5T 1R8 Canada
[b] Department of Psychiatry, University of Toronto, 250 College Street, Toronto, ON M5T 1R8 Canada
* Dr Zucker is the chair of the DSM-5 Sexual and Gender Identity Disorders Work Group.
† Corresponding author.
E-mail address: Ken_Zucker@camh.net

Child Adolesc Psychiatric Clin N Am 20 (2011) 665–680
doi:10.1016/j.chc.2011.07.006
1056-4993/11/$ – see front matter © 2011 Elsevier Inc. All rights reserved.

behaviors, along with an evaluation of the child's desire to be of the other gender (or some alternative gender that differs from the gender assigned at birth in relation to biological sex). Some clinicians, however, eschew the diagnostic label of GID (eg, to minimize stigma) and prefer alternative terms, including gender variance and transgenderism.[4] Indeed, the title of this volume is evocative, as it uses the term "gender variant" to characterize the children under consideration, perhaps with the goal of broadening the kinds of children who may come to the attention of the clinician yet, at the same time, perhaps, implying that not all of these children meet the criteria for GID or that any form of suffering that they may experience may be explained largely as a function of nonsupportive social environments, including parental nonacceptance or peer ostracism.

The clinician needs to be mindful, therefore, that these alternative terms may be, or may not be, equivalent in meaning to the intended use of the GID diagnosis. For example, the noun "variance" is defined as "the amount by which something changes or is different from something else"; the noun "variation" is defined as "a change or slight difference in condition . . . a different or distinct form or version," and the noun "variant" is defined as "a form or version that varies from other forms of the same thing."[5] One should be cognizant that, as applied to gender development, variation in gender-typed behavior is not, ipso facto, equivalent to the clinical diagnosis of GID. Indeed, it is quite likely that the omnibus term of gender variance scoops in a broader range of children than those who meet the DSM diagnostic criteria for GID.

DIAGNOSIS AND ASSESSMENT

In the development of the diagnostic criteria for GID in DSM-IV (1994),[1] the Subcommittee on Gender Identity Disorders of the American Psychiatric Association (APA) recommended that the two DSM-III (1980) and DSM-III-R (1984) diagnoses of gender identity disorder of childhood (GIDC) and transsexualism be collapsed into one overarching diagnosis, gender identity disorder (GID), with the diagnostic criteria reflecting age-related, developmental differences in clinical presentation, with separate criteria sets for children versus adolescents and adults.[6]

Box 1 shows the DSM-IV child criteria for GID. For the DSM-IV, the Subcommittee on Gender Identity Disorders reviewed the merit of altering the criteria for children to a polythetic format, in which various behavioral traits would be operationalized, from which a specified number would be required to meet the criteria for the diagnosis of GID.[6] In its final form, there were two clinical indicator (symptom) criteria. As shown in **Box 1**, Criterion A was described as "[a] strong and persistent cross-gender identification (not merely a desire for any perceived cultural advantages of being the other sex)" and a child was deemed to meet this criterion if he or she manifested at least 4 of the 5 indicators. Criterion B was described as a "[p]ersistent discomfort with his or her sex or sense of inappropriateness in the gender role of that sex" and a child was deemed to meet this criterion if he or she manifested at least 1 of 2 indicators.

Reliability and Validity

As noted elsewhere,[7] one concern about the DSM criteria for GID (in all of the editions, starting with DSM-III) is that there has been very little in the way of systematic research that documents evidence for interclinician reliability of the diagnosis. There have, however, been numerous comparative studies of the sex-typed behavior of "gender-referred" (a common pre–DSM-III term) children versus various control groups (siblings, clinical controls, and nonreferred controls), and this line of research has been used to establish the validity of the GID diagnosis. Such studies have relied on a variety of measurement approaches: item analysis from

---

Box 1
DSM-IV diagnostic criteria for gender identity disorder (child criteria)

A. A strong and persistent cross-gender identification (not merely a desire for any perceived cultural advantages of being the other sex).

In children, the disturbance is manifested by at least four (or more) of the following:

1. repeatedly stated desire to be, or insistence that he or she is, the other sex

2. in boys, preference for cross-dressing or simulating female attire; in girls, insistence on wearing only stereotypical masculine clothing

3. strong and persistent preferences for cross-sex roles in make-believe play or persistent fantasies of being the other sex

4. intense desire to participate in the stereotypical games and pastimes of the other sex

5. strong preference for playmates of the other sex.

B. Persistent discomfort with his or her sex or sense of inappropriateness in the gender role of that sex.

In children, the disturbance is manifested by any of the following: in boys, assertion that his penis or testes are disgusting or will disappear or assertion that it would be better not to have a penis, or aversion toward rough-and-tumble play and rejection of male stereotypical toys, games, and activities; in girls, rejection of urinating in a sitting position, assertion that she has or will grow a penis, or assertion that she does not want to grow breasts or menstruate, or marked aversion toward normative feminine clothing.

C. The disturbance is not concurrent with a physical intersex condition.

D. The disturbance causes clinically significant distress or impairment in social, occupational, or other important areas of functioning.

From American Psychiatric Association 2000; with permission. Only criteria for children are listed.

---

questionnaires, standardized behavioral observations, or psychometrically sound questionnaires (for a summary review of commonly used measures, see Zucker[7,8]). This line of research constitutes some of the strongest evidence for the validity of the GID diagnosis vis-á-vis the psychometric concept of "discriminant validity."

Threshold versus subthreshold comparative analyses
Within clinic-referred samples of gender-referred children, the majority have been deemed to meet the complete DSM criteria for GID based on clinician diagnosis. For example, in a cross-clinic, cross-national study of gender-referred children (total N = 488) in Toronto, Canada, and Utrecht, the Netherlands, the percentage who met the complete DSM criteria for GID was 67.0%.[9]

Some critics have expressed concern that the DSM criteria may not adequately differentiate children with GID from those children who merely show a pattern of extreme "gender nonconforming" behavior but who are not "truly" GID.[10] Interestingly, however, one analog-vignette study found that clinicians were prone to "profound underdiagnosi[is]" of GID (ie, they did not make the diagnosis even when the vignette included information that was consistent with the DSM-IV criteria as currently formulated).[11]

Given the criticism, comparative analysis of threshold versus subthreshold cases is important. First, using external measures, it can indicate whether the DSM criteria reliably distinguish between these 2 diagnostic subgroups; in other words, the central issue is one of identifying the boundary for psychiatric disorder.[12] Second, if there is evidence that a valid distinction can be made, one can evaluate whether the subgroups differ in other ways, such as variation in long-term developmental trajectories, putative etiologic factors, therapeutic considerations, and so on.

Zucker[7] reviewed the extant empirical literature that has compared threshold versus subthreshold cases using various measures of sex-typed behavior. A consistent finding has been that the threshold cases were, on average, more extreme in their cross-sex-typed behavior than the subthreshold cases. In 1 study using a parent-report questionnaire, the Gender Identity Questionnaire for Children (GIQC), Johnson and colleagues[13] found that the subthreshold group (n = 109) had a mean score that was intermediate between that of the threshold cases (n = 216) and the controls (n = 504). There was, however, clear evidence that the subthreshold group was "gender nonconforming" in that the effect size between their mean score and that of the controls was substantial (Cohen's d ranged from 1.44 to 3.28 when blocked by age groups [eg, 3 to 5 years, 5 to 6 years, etc]). In a sample of gender-referred children from the Netherlands, Cohen-Kettenis and associates[14] also found that the threshold cases (n = 114) had a significantly more deviant score on the GIQC than did the subthreshold cases (n = 42).

An important study pertaining to the threshold-subthreshold distinction was reported by Wallien and colleagues.[15] They conducted a confirmatory factor analysis (CFA) on the Gender Identity Interview for Children (GIIC), a child-informant measure of gender identity confusion, in a sample of 329 gender-referred children from Canada, 228 gender-referred children from the Netherlands, and 173 control children. The CFA documented the two-factor solution originally reported by Zucker and associates.[16] Both groups of gender-referred children had, on average, a significantly higher score on the GIIC than did the control children, indicating more gender identity confusion (Toronto-control effect size, 2.15; Amsterdam-control effect size, 3.46). More importantly, the threshold cases had a significantly higher GIIC sum score (mean, 9.58; SD, 5.70; N = 397) than did the subthreshold cases (mean, 4.68; SD, 4.18; N = 160).

Overall, these data suggest that, even within a population of gender-referred children, the DSM criteria, when used categorically (threshold vs subthreshold), significantly differentiate the behavior of the subgroups on external measures. There are, however, limitations to these kinds of analyses that should be acknowledged. For example, different combinations of the Point A and Point B criteria could (and probably did) result in a child meeting the complete criteria for GID (eg, such combinations could include children who met A1 through A5 vs A2 to A5 or even A1 and 1 of 3 combinations of A2 to A5). As well, these studies did not report how many indicators of the criteria were met for the children who were judged subthreshold for the diagnosis. Nonetheless, that in these various studies the subthreshold cases fall between that of the threshold cases and controls on external measures is consistent with the notion that there is a spectrum of gender-variant behavior, in which not all children exceed the diagnostic threshold for GID.

Predictive validity

In addition to discriminant validity, there is also some evidence of predictive validity. Wallien and Cohen-Kettenis[17] reported psychosexual follow-up data on 77 gender-referred children (59 boys, 18 girls), originally assessed at a mean age of 8.4 years (range, 5 to 12). At the time of follow-up, the mean age was 18.9 years (range, 16 to 28). Regarding gender identity at follow-up, 21 children (18 boys, 9 girls) were classified as persisters (ie, these children were still gender dysphoric and were seen clinically because of the desire for sex-reassignment [hormonal and surgical treatment]); the remaining 56 children were classified as desisters (ie, they were no longer gender-dysphoric), either based on a formal reassessment or because they had not recontacted the clinic requesting sex-reassignment. Of the 21 persisters, all had received a DSM-III-R diagnosis of GIDC at the time of assessment in childhood, compared to 37 (66.0%) of the desisters, a significant difference. On two dimensional measures of cross-gender identity, the GIQC and the GIIC, the persisters showed significantly more cross-gender behavior and gender identity confusion than the desisters. Thus, using both categorical diagnosis and dimensional measures, Wallien and Cohen-Kettenis provided some evidence for predictive validity vis-a-vis persistence versus desistance. Another follow-up study by Singh and colleagues[18] of gender-referred boys also found similar significant differences between persisters and desisters on the GIQC and GIIC.

Criticisms of the DSM-IV GID diagnosis

Since the publication of DSM-IV, there have been various critiques leveled at the GID diagnosis at it applies to children (for a detailed review, see Zucker[7]). One important criticism pertained to the revision of the Point A criterion, in which the verbalized wish to be of the other gender was collapsed with other behavioral indicators of cross-gender identification (in DSM-III and DSM-III-R, it was a distinct criterion).

Although there was empirical evidence for collapsing these indicators,[19] critics of the DSM-IV Point A criteria argued that they inappropriately condensed cross-gender identity (the desire to be of the other sex), as reflected in A1, and pervasive cross-gender role behaviors, as reflected in A2 to A5.[20] Thus, it has been claimed that the Point A criterion blurs the distinction between a child who has both a cross-gender identity and pervasive cross-gender behavior and a child who merely shows signs of pervasive cross-gendered behavior (the "gender nonconforming" or "gender-variant" child). As a result, there is the concern that children might be inappropriately diagnosed with GID simply because they meet the A2 to A5 criteria.

Toward DSM-5

The APA's Gender Identity Disorders subworkgroup for DSM-5 has provided several recommendations for modifying the current DSM criteria for GID in children (for details, see www.dsm5.org). **Box 2** shows the proposed revisions to the diagnostic criteria. The proposed changes are as follows: (1) The subworkgroup has proposed a change in the name of the diagnosis to Gender Dysphoria. This was motivated, in part, by several considerations. One consideration was that the term GID did not fully capture the "incongruence" between one's assigned gender and one's somatic sex, particularly in older children and in adolescents and adults. A second consideration was that some critics thought that eliminating the word "disorder" from the diagnostic label would reduce stigma. Third, the term "gender dysphoria," which has a rich and long history in clinical sexology,[21] was deemed to capture well the felt incongruence. (2) A 6-month duration criterion has been proposed as a lower bound, which may help clinicians rule out symptoms of a transient nature.[22] (3) The subworkgroup has recommended that the Point A and B criteria in DSM-IV be collapsed into 1 criterion set, based on the view that one underlying factor best captures the phenomenology of gender dysphoria. (4) There has been some minor wording changes to the clinical indicators. (5) Subtyping as a function of the presence versus absence of a disorder of sex development (DSD) (physical intersex conditions) has been proposed, since there is good clinical evidence that individuals with a DSD can experience gender dysphoria.[23] The presence of a DSD is likely a predisposing factor that individuals

---

Box 2
Proposed DSM-5 diagnostic criteria for gender dysphoria in children

A. A marked incongruence between one's experienced/expressed gender and assigned gender, of at least 6 months duration, as manifested by at least 6 of the following indicators (including A1):

  1. a strong desire to be of the other gender or an insistence that he or she is the other gender (or some alternative gender different from one's assigned gender)

  2. in boys, a strong preference for cross-dressing or simulating female attire; in girls, a strong preference for wearing only typical masculine clothing and a strong resistance to the wearing of typical feminine clothing

  3. a strong preference for cross-gender roles in make-believe or fantasy play

  4. a strong preference for the toys, games, or activities typical of the other gender

  5. a strong preference for playmates of the other gender

  6. in boys, a strong rejection of typically masculine toys, games, and activities and a strong avoidance of rough-and-tumble play; in girls, a strong rejection of typically feminine toys, games, and activities

  7. a strong dislike of one's sexual anatomy

  8. a strong desire for the primary and/or secondary sex characteristics that match one's experienced gender.

B. The condition is associated with clinically significant distress or impairment in social, occupational, or other important areas of functioning, or with a significantly increased risk of suffering, such as distress or disability.

Subtypes

With a disorder of sex development

Without a disorder of sex development

Data from American Psychiatric Association. DSM-5: the Future of Psychiatric Diagnosis. Available at www.dsm5.org. Accessed may 28, 2011.

---

without a DSD do not share.[24] (6) To avoid the possibility of overdiagnosing children with extreme gender-variant behavior, the desire to be of the other gender (A1) has been proposed as a necessary symptom. As reviewed by Zucker,[7] a reanalysis of secondary data sets was consistent with the hypothesis that the presence of A1 would likely reduce the possibility of overdiagnosis based on the presence of surface behaviors that reflect cross-gender identification per se but not necessarily gender dysphoria.

Regarding the A1 criterion, there is, however, an important change in wording. It can be seen in **Box 2** that the persistent desire to be of the other gender does not explicitly require that this be verbalized and, therefore, allows the clinician latitude in inferring it based on other clinical evidence. For example, some clinicians have suggested that in unaccepting environments some children may inhibit their verbalized expression to be of the other gender, but that the desire may become more manifest in a more accepting environment (eg, after rapport is established with a clinician).

Quantitative Assessment of Sex-Typed Behavior

Over the years, several research teams have reported on various sex-typed measures that can be used in the assessment of gender variance.[8] **Table 1** shows the sex-typed assessment protocol that has been developed in my own clinic, with modifications, over a 35-year period.

Table 1	
Sex-typed assessment protocol	
Test/Task/Questionnaire	**Reference**
Child Measures	
Draw-a-Person test	Zucker and colleagues[36]
Free Play Task	Zucker and colleagues[37]
Playmate and Play Style Preferences Structured Interview	Fridell and colleagues[38]
Color Preference Task	Chiu and colleagues[39]
Gender Constancy Tasks	Zucker and colleagues[40]
Gender Identity Interview for Children	Wallien and colleagues,[15] Zucker and colleagues[16]
Rorschach	Zucker and colleagues[41]
Parent Measures	
Temperament Questionnaire	Zucker and Bradley[25]
Games Inventory	Bates and Bentler[42]
Gender Identity Questionnaire for Children	Johnson and colleagues[13]

Note. For other sex-typed measures that can be used with gender variant children, see Zucker.[8]

Some measures are relatively brief and can be easily used by the practicing clinician. Other measures are more difficult to use outside of a specialized research unit, since standard sets of stimuli (eg, certain toys and dress-up apparel) are required. In general, however, the use of these measures can compliment the more routine clinical interview and can provide a more dimensionalized picture of the child's clinical presentation.

Two examples will be provided. The parent-report GIQC[13] provides a mean score that dimensionalizes the degree of a child's cross-gender behavior and, with the use of standard deviation scores, can identify where an individual child's score lies compared to other gender-referred children of a similar age as well as to same-age control children. Johnson and associates[13] also suggested a cutoff score to identify "caseness." Because this scale appears to be relatively impervious to age effects, it is possible to track an individual child's score over time, with comparison to group data of both GID children and control children.

Figures 1–3 provide examples of the GIQC for three children. Case 93 (see **Fig. 1**) was an 8-year-old girl (IQ = 94) at the baseline assessment, at which time she met the DSM-III-R criteria for GID. At baseline, her GIQC score was more extreme than that of other children referred for gender identity issues at age 8 and considerably more extreme than that of 8-year-old control children. Apart from the GID, this youngster had a myriad of other socioemotional problems, including posttraumatic stress disorder and oppositional-defiant disorder, and had been in the care of child protection services since the age of 5. At a 1-year follow-up, her mean GIQC score was similar to that of other children referred for gender identity issues at age 9 but considerably more extreme than that of 9-year-old control children. At a second follow-up at the age of 12, her mean GIQC was more extreme than that of other children referred for gender identity issues at age 12 and considerably more extreme than that of 12-year-old control children. Thus, this youngster showed very little change in her mean GIQC scores from baseline to follow-up. At the age of 23 years, this patient showed persistent gender dysphoria and had a gynephilic sexual orientation (in relation to birth sex).

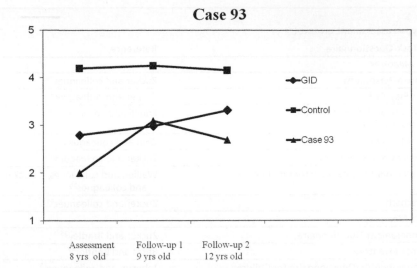

Fig. 1. Maternal ratings on the Gender Identity Questionnaire for Children.[13] Vertical axis represents the 5-point response scale. A lower score indicates more cross-gender behavior/ less same-gender behavior. *Data from* Johnson LL, Bradley SJ, Birkenfeld-Adams AS, et al. A parent-report Gender Identity Questionnaire for Children. Arch Sex Behav 2004;33:105–16.

Case 343 (see **Fig. 2**) was an 8-year-old boy (IQ = 81) at the baseline assessment, at which time he met the DSM-IV criteria for GID. At baseline, his GIQC score was more extreme than that of other children referred for gender identity issues at age 8 and considerably more extreme than that of 8-year-old control children. Apart from the GID, this youngster had a variety of other socioemotional problems and met

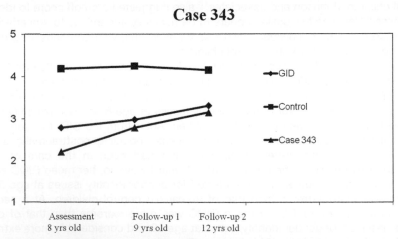

Fig. 2. Maternal ratings on the Gender Identity Questionnaire for Children.[13] Vertical axis represents the 5-point response scale. A lower score indicates more cross-gender behavior/ less same-gender behavior. *Data from* Johnson LL, Bradley SJ, Birkenfeld-Adams AS, et al. A parent-report Gender Identity Questionnaire for Children. Arch Sex Behav 2004;33:105–16.

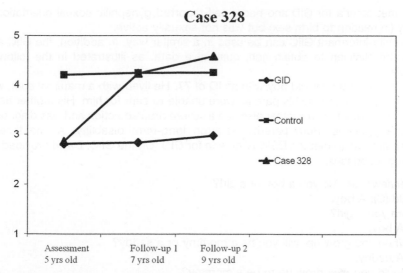

Fig. 3. Maternal ratings on the Gender Identity Questionnaire for Children.[13] Vertical axis represents the 5-point response scale. A lower score indicates more cross-gender behavior/less same-gender behavior. *Data from* Johnson LL, Bradley SJ, Birkenfeld-Adams AS, et al. A parent-report Gender Identity Questionnaire for Children. Arch Sex Behav 2004;33:105–16.

criteria for oppositional-defiant disorder, generalized anxiety disorder, and separation anxiety disorder. The parents did not want to address their son's gender identity issues in therapy but, rather, wanted to work on the other difficulties that he had been experiencing. Thus, over the course of 3 years of weekly therapy (parent counseling and individual child therapy), the treatment of this youngster focused on these other issues but not on his gender-related behavior. At a 1-year follow-up, his mean GIQC score was similar to that of other children referred for gender identity issues at age 9 but considerably more extreme than that of 9-year-old control children. At a second follow-up at the age of 12, his mean GIQC was more extreme than that of other children referred for gender identity issues at age 12 and considerably more extreme than that of 12-year-old control children. Thus, this youngster showed very little change in his mean GIQC scores from baseline to follow-up. At the age of 20 years, this patient no longer met criteria for GID and had a self-reported androphilic sexual orientation (in relation to birth sex).

Case 328 (see **Fig. 3**) was a 5-year-old boy (IQ = 104) at the baseline assessment, at which time he met the DSM-IV criteria for GID. At baseline, his GIQC score was similar to that of other children referred for gender identity issues at age 5 and considerably more extreme than that of 5-year-old control children. Apart from the GID, this youngster was shy and extremely anxious. In the course of 39 months of individual therapy (101 sessions) and parent counseling (82 sessions), both the gender identity issues and the anxiety were foci of intervention. At the age of 7, his mean GIQC score was considerably less than that of other children referred for gender identity issues at age 7 but similar to that of 7-year-old control children. At a second follow-up at the age of 9, his mean GIQC was considerably less than that of other children referred for gender identity issues at age 9, but similar to that of 9-year-old control children. Thus, this youngster showed a significant change in his mean GIQC scores from baseline to follow-up. At the age of 18 years, this patient no longer met criteria for GID and had a self-reported gynephilic sexual orientation in fantasy (in relation to birth sex) but was not sexually active.

The child-informant GIIC can be used in a similar way. In addition, the GIIC also allows the clinician to obtain rich, qualitative data, as illustrated in the following example:

David was an 8-year-old boy with an IQ of 77. He lived with a maternal aunt, who was raising him because his parents were unable to care for him. His mother had a severe drug addiction; his father also had a severe drug addiction and was diagnosed with schizophrenia. Both parents were on long-term disability. At the time of assessment, David met the DSM-IV criteria for GID. On the GIIC, David provided the following responses:

> Interviewer (I): Are you a boy or a girl?
> Child (C): A boy.
> I: Are you a girl?
> C: A boy.
> I: When you grow up, will you be a mommy or a saddy?
> C: A daddy.
> I: Could you ever grow up to be a mommy?
> C: No.
> I: Are there any good things about being a boy?
> C: Yes . . . It's fun. That's it . . . that's all I know about boys.
> I: Are there any things that you don't like about being a boy?
> C: Yes . . . I don't like the penis. It's disgusting for me. I don't like how boys react . . . I don't like how they play, like they mess up a lot.
> I: Do you think it is better to be a boy or a girl?
> C: Girl . . . because they're cute. They don't mess up.
> I: In your mind, do you ever think that you would like to be a girl?
> C: Yes.
> I: Can you tell me why?
> C: What I don't like is when I just mess up and stuff . . . It means boys like to mess up a lot.
> I: Do you ever feel more like a girl than like a boy?
> C: Yes . . . well, I don't like how boys react . . .
> I: You know what dreams are, right? Well, when you dream at night, are you ever in the dream?
> C: Yes.
> I: In your dreams, are you a boy, a girl, or sometimes a boy and sometimes a girl?
> C: Girl.
> I: Tell me about that.
> C: Once I was a robber girl. The funnest [sic] dream that happened was when I was 5 years old. It was a nightmare. It was so scary.
> I: Do you ever think that you really are a girl?
> C: Yes.
> I: Tell me more about that.
> C: I don't know . . . always.

Another easy-to-use measure, especially for the clinician in a private practice setting, is the Draw-a-Person test (**Table 1**), a projective task. When asked to "draw a person," most children draw first a child that matches their birth sex. In contrast, children with gender identity issues are much more likely to draw a person of the other sex. A common interpretation of this pattern is that it reflects the gender with which

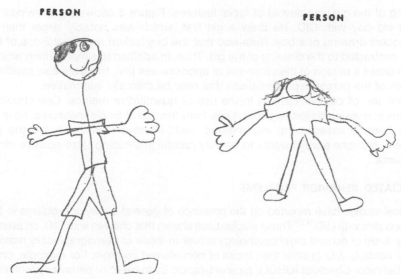

Fig. 4. Human figure drawings by a 6-year-old girl with gender identity disorder.

the child more strongly identifies. **Figures 4** and **5** provide 2 examples. **Figure 4** shows the drawings of a 6-year-old girl with GID. She drew a boy first, which was taller than her subsequent drawing of a girl, which she identified as "me having a bad hair day." Note also that the boy drawing had detailed facial features, but that the

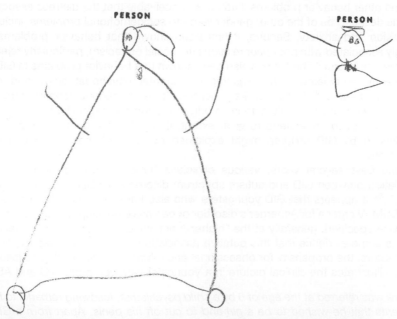

Fig. 5. Human figure drawings by a 5-year-old boy with gender identity disorder.

drawing of the girl was devoid of facial features. **Figure 5** shows the drawings of a 5-year-old boy with GID. He drew a girl first, which was notably larger than the subsequent drawing of a boy. Note also that the boy lacked representations of feet, which contrasted to the drawing of the girl. Thus, in addition to simply noting whether a child draws a person of the same-sex or opposite-sex first, there are also qualitative features of the person representations that may be clinically informative.

There are, of course, caveats in the use of quantitative metrics. One should be cautious in drawing definitive conclusions from the use of single measures. As in any comprehensive assessment, multimethod, multi-informant protocols are the gold standard, and one always wants to be very careful in avoiding false-positive clinical judgments.

ASSOCIATED BEHAVIOR PROBLEMS

Empirical studies have reported on the presence of general behavior problems in both boys and girls with GID.[9,25] These studies have shown that children with GID, on average, display levels of general psychopathology similar to those of demographically matched clinical controls and greater than those of nonreferred controls. For example, on the Child Behavior Checklist (CBCL), a parent-report instrument of behavior problems,[26] children with GID have been shown to display behavior problems at a level comparable to the clinic-referred standardization sample[25] and the Cohen-Kettenis and colleagues[9] study was the first to demonstrate similar rates of behavior problems cross-nationally. Boys with GID generally show more internalizing than externalizing problems on the CBCL, whereas internalizing and externalizing problems are more evenly distributed among girls with GID. Some boys with GID have also been shown to manifest traits of separation anxiety disorder.[27,28] One study that used a categorical structured diagnostic interview schedule found that 52% of GID children (total N = 120) met criteria for at least one other psychiatric diagnosis.[29]

There are several ways in which one might be consider the association between GID and other behavior problems. First, it is conceivable that the distress associated with the desire to be of the other gender leads to socioemotional problems, including depression and anxiety. Second, it has been shown that behavior problems are strongly associated with poor peer relations (ie, social ostracism, particularly rejection by same-sex peers).[9] Third, it has also been shown that behavior problems in GID are significantly associated with measures of parental psychopathology and other general risk factors.[30] Thus, it is likely that the causes of general behavior problems in children with GID are multifactorial in origin. A good clinical evaluation, therefore, should attempt to understand to what extent, if any, the socioemotional problems experienced by GID children might explained by each of these aforementioned parameters.

In the past several years, various clinicians have reported on a new, novel association between GID and autism spectrum disorders (ASDs), including 1 group study.[31,32] It appears that GID youngsters who also have an ASD are most likely to meet DSM-IV criteria for Asperger's disorder or pervasive developmental disorder not otherwise specified, generally at the "higher-functioning" end of the ASD spectrum. There is some evidence that this putative association may be explained by, among other factors, the propensity for obsessional and restricted interests.[33] The following vignette illustrates the clinical picture in a youngster with comorbid GID and ASD:

Frank was referred at the age of 5 by a child psychiatrist, following remarks to his parents that he wished to be a girl and to cut off his penis. Apart from a GID, Frank had a number of socioemotional difficulties, including persistent and pervasive struggles with self-regulation, behavioral rigidity, obsessive behaviors, anxiety, and poor social functioning. In our assessment, we concluded that he met criteria for Asperger's disorder. Play therapy was initiated to help explore Frank's gender dysphoria. As appropriate, additional therapeutic strategies were drawn upon in order to support the development of self-regulation (eg, with regard to sexualized behavior directed toward the therapist, temper tantrums), social skills, and the management of areas of obsessive focus. In the therapeutic context, struggles with the parent-child relationship, self-concept, peer relations, and anger and guilt were consistent themes. Over the course of 4 years in therapy, Frank evidenced a strong tendency toward obsessions/restricted interests (eg, trains, airports, certain television shows, and book series), with each lasting between 3 to 6 months in duration. The gender-related preoccupation stood out in terms of its relationship to identity. The gender dysphoria began to wane around age 7 and little in the way of GID symptoms was seen in the therapeutic context for the past 18 months. At age 9 years, in the 112th therapy session, Frank initiated discussion about his history of obsessions/restricted interests. He requested that his therapist write out each of his areas of interest (in chronologic order) and he proceeded to summarize the "rationale" behind each. Early in the list, he placed his preoccupation with cross-gender materials. Frank paused on this area and reflected it had carried special meaning for him. He went on to say that this may have been more than just an interest in this topic area and that, in fact, he had wanted to be a girl. He reflected on the reinforcing aspects of many of the feminine interests and behaviors (eg, the feeling of pretend long hair, how "beautiful" things looked, etc), with a focus on the associated visual and tactile stimulation. When asked about his understanding of his involvement in therapy, starting at age 5 years, Frank reflected that his parents may have been concerned about his desire to be a girl, as they knew that he was "really a boy." He recalled his parent's efforts to curtail his cross-gender behaviors by limiting his time and access. He discussed his belief that this was not the right approach, and that he should have just been allowed him to grow out of this interest, as he had all of the previous and subsequent ones. In reflecting on his development of gender dysphoria, Frank discussed his experience of bullying from peers for his gender atypical areas of interest. He speculated that, in many ways, his desire to become a girl may have been an effort to avoid the bullying from peers. Frank again reiterated the very reinforcing aspects of many of his female-typical interests. Finally, he reflected on his negative feeling about himself and his behavior and we considered his gender dysphoria as an effort to cope with these feelings. Frank continues to demonstrate a tendency toward preoccupations but, at present, has no symptoms characteristic of GID. He continues to benefit from therapeutic support for self-regulation, social skills, and management of his restricted interests/preoccupations.

SUMMARY

Subsequent to the two prior volumes of *Child and Adolescent Psychiatric Clinics of North America* that have focused on sex and gender issues,[34,35] there have continued to be solid advances in the development of assessment procedures for children who are in the gender-variant spectrum. In recent years, largely due to increased media exposure, there is a much greater public awareness of the complexities that gender-variant children encounter in their day-to-day lives. The contemporary clinician is, therefore, probably more likely to encounter such children in the mental health system. It is hoped that the assessment options summarized here will be of use in providing best-practice care.

REFERENCES

1. American Psychiatric Association. Diagnostic and statistical manual of mental disorders. 4th edition, text revision. Washington, DC: American Psychiatric Association; 2000.
2. Ruble DN, Martin CL, Berenbaum SA. Gender development. In: Damon W, Lerner RM, series editors, and Eisenberg N, volume editor. Handbook of child psychology. 6th edition, vol. 3: social, emotional, and personality development. New York: Wiley; 2010. p. 858–932.
3. Blakemore JEO, Berenbaum SA, Liben LS. Gender development. New York: Psychology Press; 2009.
4. Pleak RR. Ethical issues in diagnosing and treating gender-dysphoric children and adolescents. In: Rottnek M, editor. Sissies & tomboys: gender nonconformity & homosexual childhood. New York: New York University Press; 1999. p. 44–51.
5. Soanes C, editor. Oxford dictionary of current English. 3rd edition. New York: Oxford University Press; 2001.
6. Bradley SJ, Blanchard R, Coates S, et al. Interim report of the DSM-IV Subcommittee on Gender Identity Disorders. Arch Sex Behav 1991;20:333–43.
7. Zucker KJ. The DSM diagnostic criteria for gender identity disorder in children. Arch Sex Behav 2010;39:477–98.
8. Zucker KJ. Measurement of psychosexual differentiation. Arch Sex Behav 2005;34: 375–88.
9. Cohen-Kettenis PT, Owen A, Kaijser VG, et al. Demographic characteristics, social competence, and behavior problems in children with gender identity disorder: a cross-national, cross-clinic comparative analysis. J Abnorm Child Psychol 2003;31: 41–53.
10. Corbett K. Homosexual boyhood: notes on girlyboys. Gender Psychoanalysis 1996; 1:429–61.
11. Ehrbar RD, Witty MC, Ehrbar HG, et al. Clinician judgment in the diagnosis of gender identity disorder in children. J Sex Marital Ther 2008;34:385–412.
12. Kendler KS. Setting boundaries for psychiatric disorders [editorial]. Am J Psychiatry 1999;156:1845–8.
13. Johnson LL, Bradley SJ, Birkenfeld-Adams AS, et al. A parent-report Gender Identity Questionnaire for Children. Arch Sex Behav 2004;33:105–16.
14. Cohen-Kettenis PT, Wallien M, Johnson LL, et al. A parent-report Gender Identity Questionnaire for Children: a cross-national, cross-clinic comparative analysis. Clin Child Psychol Psychiatry 2006;11:397–405.
15. Wallien MSC, Quilty LC, Steensma TD, et al. Cross-national replication of the Gender Identity Interview for Children. J Pers Assess 2009;91:545–52.
16. Zucker KJ, Bradley SJ, Lowry Sullivan CB, et al. A gender identity interview for children. J Pers Assess 1993;61:443–56.
17. Wallien MSC, Cohen-Kettenis PT. Psychosexual outcome of gender-dysphoric children. J Am Acad Child Adolesc Psychiatry 2008;47:1413–23.
18. Singh D, Bradley SJ, Zucker KJ. A follow-up study of boys with gender identity disorder. Presented at the University of Lethbridge Workshop, The Puzzle of Sexual Orientation: What Is It and How Does It Work? Lethbridge, Alberta, Canada, June 2010.
19. Zucker KJ, Green R, Bradley SJ, et al. Gender identity disorder of childhood: diagnostic issues. In: Widiger TA, Frances AJ, Pincus HA, et al, editors. DSM-IV

sourcebook, vol. 4. Washington, DC: American Psychiatric Association; 1998. p. 503–12.

20. Bartlett NH, Vasey PL, Bukowski WM. Is gender identity disorder in children a mental disorder? Sex Roles 2000;43:753–85.

21. Fisk N. Gender dysphoria syndrome (the how, what, and why of a disease). In: Laub D, Gandy P, editors. Proceedings of the Second Interdisciplinary Symposium on Gender Dysphoria Syndrome. Palo Alto (CA): Stanford University Press, 1973. p. 7–14.

22. Linday LA. Maternal reports of pregnancy, genital, and related fantasies in preschool and kindergarten children. J Am Acad Child Adolesc Psychiatry 1994;33:416–23.

23. Richter-Appelt H, Sandberg DE. Should disorders of sex development be an exclusion criterion for gender identity disorder in DSM 5? Int J Transgenderism 2010;12: 94–9.

24. Meyer-Bahlburg HFL. Intersexuality and the diagnosis of gender identity disorder. Arch Sex Behav 1994;23:21–40.

25. Zucker KJ, Bradley SJ. Gender identity disorder and psychosexual problems in children and adolescents. New York: Guilford Press; 1995.

26. Achenbach TM, Edelbrock C. Manual for the Child Behavior Checklist and Revised Child Behavior Profile. Burlington (VT): University of Vermont, Department of Psychiatry; 1983.

27. Coates S, Person ES. Extreme boyhood femininity: isolated behavior or pervasive disorder? J Am Acad Child Psychiatry 1985;24:702–9.

28. Zucker KJ, Bradley SJ, Lowry Sullivan CB. Traits of separation anxiety in boys with gender identity disorder. J Am Acad Child Adolesc Psychiatry 1996;35:791–8.

29. Wallien MSC, Swaab H, Cohen-Kettenis PT. Psychiatric comorbidity among children with gender identity disorder. J Am Acad Child Adolesc Psychiatry 2007;46:1307–14.

30. Zucker KJ. Associated psychopathology in children and adolescents with gender identity disorder. In: Meyer-Bahlburg HFL, chair, From mental disorder to iatrogenic hypogonadism: dilemmas in conceptualizing gender identity disorder (GID) as a psychiatric condition. Symposium presented at the meeting of the American Academy of Child and Adolescent Psychiatry, Chicago, October 2008.

31. Williams PG, Allard AM, Sears L. Case study: cross-gender preoccupations with two male children with autism. J Autism Dev Disord 1996;26:635–42.

32. de Vries ALC, Noens IL, Cohen-Kettenis PT, et al. Autism spectrum disorders in gender dysphoric children and adolescents. J Autism Dev Disord 2010;40:930–6.

33. Postema L, Wood H, Singh D, et al. Do children with gender identity disorder have intense/obsessional interests? A preliminary study. Paper presented at the meeting of the World Professional Association for Transgender Health. Atlanta, Georgia, September 2011.

34. Zucker KJ, Green R. Psychological and familial aspects of gender identity disorder. Child Adolesc Psychiatr Clin N Am 1993;2:513–42.

35. Zucker KJ. Gender identity development and issues. Child Adolesc Psychiatr Clin N Am 2004;13:551–68.

36. Zucker KJ, Finegan JK, Doering RW, et al. Human figure drawings of gender-problem children: a comparison to sibling, psychiatric, and normal controls. J Abnorm Child Psychol 1983;11:287–98.

37. Zucker KJ, Doering RW, Bradley SJ, et al. Sex-typed play in gender-disturbed children: a comparison to sibling and psychiatric controls. Arch Sex Behav 1982;11: 309–21.

38. Fridell SR, Owen-Anderson A, Johnson LL, et al. The Playmate and Play Style Preferences Structured Interview: a comparison of children with gender identity disorder and controls. Arch Sex Behav 2006;35:729–37.
39. Chiu SW, Gervan S, Fairbrother C, et al. Sex-dimorphic color preference in children with gender identity disorder: a comparison to clinical and community controls. Sex Roles 2006;55:385–95.
40. Zucker KJ, Bradley SJ, Kuksis M, et al. Gender constancy judgments in children with gender identity disorder: evidence for a developmental lag. Arch Sex Behav 1999;28: 475–502.
41. Zucker KJ, Lozinski JA, Bradley SJ, et al. Sex-typed responses in the Rorschach protocols of children with gender identity disorder. J Pers Assess 1992;58:295–310.
42. Bates JE, Bentler PM. Play activities of normal and effeminate boys. Dev Psychol 1973;9:20–7.

Female-to-Male Transgender Adolescents

Sarah E. Herbert, MD, MSW

KEYWORDS

• Adolescent • Female-to-male • Gender identity
• Transgender

This article focuses on considerations for natal females who present in the adolescent years with concerns related to their gender. They may be individuals previously evaluated in their childhood years who have persisted with gender variance or gender identity disorder (GID) in DSM-IV,[1] or they may be individuals presenting for the first time in their adolescent years. The article discusses how to assess adolescents who come for evaluation and what treatments and other resources are available for them and their families. Where there seem to be differences between boys and girls with gender identity issues, they will be noted.

DEVELOPMENTAL CONSIDERATIONS

One of the most perplexing challenges facing clinicians who work with gender-variant children is the issue of who will persist and who will desist in the desire or feeling of being the gender opposite to the natal sex. As challenging as it is to have a gender-variant child, parents often articulate the desire to at least know whether their child will persist or desist, so they can be prepared for the outcome. If the child showed all signs of persisting, plans could be made for how to handle pubertal development and the teenaged years ahead of time. If they knew their child would desist in their identification with the opposite natal sex, then they could prepare for that outcome.

What do we know about the longitudinal outcome for girls who are gender dysphoric? There are few studies that provide longitudinal follow-up of girls referred for evaluation of gender identity issues in childhood. Most studies look retrospectively at female-to-male (FTM) adults who discuss experiences from their childhood and adolescent years.[2–4]

There are 2 studies of children evaluated in childhood that afford us some longitudinal follow-up on girls with gender dysphoria. The data from the gender clinic in The Netherlands suggest that gender dysphoric girls referred in childhood are less likely to remit than boys.[5] In that study, of 77 children referred in childhood, only 18

Morehouse School of Medicine, Department of Psychiatry and Behavioral Sciences, 41-A Lenox Pointe NE, Atlanta, GA 30324, USA
E-mail address: saraheherbert@comcast.net

Child Adolesc Psychiatric Clin N Am 20 (2011) 681–688
doi:10.1016/j.chc.2011.08.005
1056-4993/11/$ – see front matter © 2011 Published by Elsevier Inc.

were girls, and 14 consented to follow-up. Surprisingly, 9 girls (64%) persisted with gender dysphoria and 5 girls desisted, a higher percentage of persistence than for the boys at follow-up.[5] Almost all of the female subjects (13 of the 14) for whom there was follow-up data met full criteria for GID at the time of initial assessment; only 1 was subthreshold for this diagnosis. All of the persisting girls had a homosexual or bisexual orientation, and all of the desisting girls reported a heterosexual orientation. In contrast, a study from the gender clinic in Toronto, Canada, that included 25 girls evaluated in childhood found very different results. At the initial assessment, 60% met criteria for GID, and 40% were subthreshold for this diagnosis.[6] At follow-up, only 12% (3 girls) were judged to have GID or gender dysphoria, a much different rate of persistence compared with the Dutch study. In the Canadian study, 88% (22 subjects) reported no distress with their female gender identity at follow-up. When sexual orientation was assessed, 32% were homosexual or bisexual in fantasy, 23% homosexual or bisexual in behavior, and 20% identified themselves as homosexual or bisexual.

Given the current state of our knowledge, it is difficult to predict with any certainty who will persist or desist. It is generally accepted that the children who persist with GID into their teens are the ones who were most extreme in their gender nonconforming behavior and feelings in childhood. If the GID is present in the adolescent years, it is also far more likely to persist than is the case for those who manifest this in childhood.[7] Adolescents who both persist and desist in cross-gender identity consider the ages 10 to 13 to be crucial in their perception of the continuing or diminishing of their childhood gender dysphoria.[8]

ASSESSMENT OF THE ADOLESCENT WITH GENDER IDENTITY CONCERNS

What issues does a mental health clinician want to address in the evaluation of a natal female adolescent with concerns about gender? To make as complete an evaluation as possible, the adolescent as well as the parents or guardians must be interviewed. Information regarding the adolescent's early psychosexual development will be important. How early did this adolescent show signs of gender variance? What were her preferences for toys, clothing, games, and peers? What comments did she make when younger about her name, her assigned sex, her body? Did she ask to be called by a male name? Did she insist on wearing typical boys' clothing? Did she think she would grow up to be a man or a daddy? What roles did she take in fantasy play with peers? Would she wear a girl's bathing suit in the summer or insist on going without a top? Have her preferences changed over time—has she become more gender nonconforming or less so?

Interviewing the adolescent alone also provides important information regarding gender issues. Does this adolescent present as male, female, or in-between? What has been her reaction to pubertal development? Is there disgust at breast development and menstruation, or has she become more accepting of changes in her body? Is her clothing masculine, are her breasts bound, is there use of something to make it appear the individual has male genitals? Is there use of a male or gender-neutral name? Is there refusal to use bathrooms associated with her biological sex? Is there refusal to change clothes for physical education in the girls' locker room? How are peer relationships? Is this adolescent well-liked and accepted, or isolated, withdrawn, or bullied? Is there any romantic interest in having a girlfriend or boyfriend? Has there been any dating? What do the teenager's sexual fantasies involve? What sexual experiences have there been? How does this person define his or her sexual orientation? Is the teen at risk for sexually transmitted diseases, including HIV?[9]

There are a number of ways in which transgender adolescents may identify themselves, and these may change over time. We may want to ask whether this adolescent sees himself or herself as a masculine female, as a male born into the wrong body, or somewhere in between. There are many examples of FTM adults who initially identified as masculine girls and women, but later felt their identity to be male, and made a successful transition to male. We may also see youth who resist labeling themselves, or may identify as gender-queer. Diamond and Butterworth[10] discussed dynamic links between questioning gender and sexual identity based on biological female subjects followed over a period of 10 years. They speculate that dichotomous models of gender identity may fail to capture the complexity, diversity, and fluidity of the transgender experience in the same way that there is now recognition that patterns of same-sex and other-sex desire show more fluidity and complexity than was previously recognized. Attempts to develop stage models of transsexual identity formation may be helpful in understanding individual patients, but they have some of the same limitations that models of homosexual identity formation do. They assume the ultimate and healthy resolution is acceptance of an unambiguous male identity and do not take into account cultural variations in concepts of identity or sexual orientation.[11,12]

Significant religious or cultural views of transgenderism and/or homosexuality are important to ask about and understand in evaluating transgender adolescents and their families.[13] Gender variance may be regarded differently depending on the cultural or religious beliefs of the adolescent or family.[14] Dissonance between the family and an adolescent on these issues can result in abuse, rejection, and/or fear. Some transgender youth have been told to leave the family home (and hence become throwaways, rather than runaways), or denied living and/or school and college expenses if they persist in their gender nonconforming behaviors.

Although gender issues definitely put an individual at risk, it is important for the clinician to ascertain how well this adolescent is adapting despite the gender variance. Is this transboy or adolescent with gender issues still able to achieve academically or in other ways, such as creatively or vocationally? Does s/he have friends, a romantic interest, or partner? Has s/he been able to maintain relationships with family members, and to have their support despite being different from the girl the parents had expected? Are there other individuals or community organizations from which this adolescent has garnered support and encouragement? Is their support and encouragement from the primary care physician?[15]

The 27-item gender identity/gender dysphoria questionnaire for adolescents and adults[16] is a validated instrument that can be used with adolescents or used as a guide to assist clinicians in questions that they may want to ask during the gender evaluation. The questions are the same for adolescents and adults except for the word girl or boy being substituted for woman or man in the adult version.

A composite example from teens who have been previously evaluated and treated is illustrated below.

Casey was a 15-year-old natal female whose parents said she had always been a "tomboy." She was a very active preschooler who loved playing with her older brother's toys and never seemed to show much interest in more stereotypically feminine activities and toys such as dolls or playhouses. Once she was old enough to articulate what she wanted to wear her mother could not get her to put on a dress. Instead, the family compromised when she agreed to dress up for church on Sundays by wearing khaki pants and an Oxford cloth shirt. She was a superb soccer player who played on a boys' team until this was no longer possible in late elementary school. Middle school was a more difficult experience for Casey. While she previously had some good friends in elementary school (although they were more likely to be boys than girls), she seemed to withdraw socially the older she got. Instead of playing sports after school, she would come home and close herself in her room, seeming to be quite irritable if anyone came to the door. The parents realized that Casey's darker moods seemed to begin with puberty, but attributed them initially to hormonal shifts that occur for all teenage girls. Casey's family expected that she would outgrow her tomboy phase, and once she started developing secondary sex characteristics they had expected that she would naturally become more feminine. Extended family members were putting more pressure on Casey's parents to make her to dress "like a 15-year-old girl." However, Casey was different: She persisted in wearing masculine-looking clothing that was big and baggy, clearly hiding any aspects of her body that seemed to indicate she was a girl. Casey would not wear any bra except for a sports bra that seemed to flatten her chest. When her mother walked into her bedroom 1 day unexpectedly, she found that Casey had wrapped her chest tightly with an Ace bandage and was in the process of stuffing a pair of socks into jockey shorts that must have belonged to her older brother. At this point, the parents realized this was more than a prolonged tomboy phase and sought help to determine what was going on with their daughter. They wanted to know if this meant their daughter was a lesbian or "worse, is she transgender?"

When Casey was interviewed, she was able with some patient questioning to describe her long-standing issues with gender identity. Although her parents knew of her lack of interest in stereotypically feminine toys, activities, and dress, she had not shared with them her intense distress about not being a boy. Nor had she been able to tell them how she felt so betrayed by her body developing in what she felt was a completely wrong direction. She could not stand having breasts and was mortified by the experience of menstruation. Casey did have some romantic interest in a female peer, but had not pursued it any further than kissing. She knew that boys were her friends, and that her romantic interests were directed toward girls. That made her feel like she must be a lesbian, but was puzzled because she didn't think she felt the way she thought lesbians did, although she wasn't sure about this.

MENTAL HEALTH ISSUES THAT PUT THE ADOLESCENT AT RISK

Peer rejection can be a major issue for the child or adolescent with gender nonconformity. Parents report that their children with gender variance have poorer social relationships than their siblings. A recent study from the Dutch gender clinic revealed that gender-referred girls were more accepted by male than by female classmates and had significantly more male and fewer female friends.[17] Unlike the gender-referred boys who were rejected by other boys, however, the gender-referred girls were not rejected by female classmates. There is some speculation that girls with gender nonconformity experience more difficulty around puberty when there is the societal expectation that they will give up their tomboy status.

It is clear that the adolescent years may be ones of turmoil for transgender teens. However, much of the data to support this comes from retrospective accounts of those years by adult transgender individuals.[18–20] Studies that have reported on mental health issues in gender-dysphoric children diagnosed before puberty have described some evidence of psychological problems. Fifty percent of children referred to the Dutch gender clinic had greater than or equal to 1 associated disorder, with 31% having an anxiety disorder.[21] However, their comparison group of children referred to a clinic for the diagnosis of attention deficit hyperactivity disorder had an even higher rate of comorbidity at 60%, and 34% of those children had an anxiety disorder. The differences in comorbidity between children with attention deficit hyperactivity disorder and GID were not significant. Children in a cross-national study using the Achenbach Child Behavior Checklist[22] found behavioral problems in the clinical range for girls and boys in samples from both The Netherlands and Canada, but this study did not formally diagnose the behavioral problems.[23]

WHAT DO STUDIES OF MENTAL HEALTH ISSUES IN CURRENT TRANSGENDER ADOLESCENTS TELL US?

Anxiety and depressive disorders are thought to be common among transgender youth. The anxiety may be related to real or perceived rejection, hostility, and abuse owing to the teen's transgender status, or fear of being "read" or discovered if the teen has had some success passing as the opposite sex. Examples of transgender teens who have committed suicide or been killed owing to gender nonconformity or transgender status abound in the media. Although society seems to have more tolerance for females who want to be males, there are examples of intolerance and abuse for girls who present themselves as boys. Brandon Teena's story of being raped and murdered was made into a popular 1999 film *Boys Don't Cry*,[24] based on the 1998 documentary *The Brandon Teena Story*.[25] Daphne Scholinski's memoir, *The Last Time I Wore a Dress*, chronicled her treatment at the hands of mental health professionals seeking to alter her gender nonconformity in the settings of a mental hospital and residential treatment facility.[26] A *New York Times Magazine* article in 2002 documented the struggles of a 13-year-old FTM teen.[27]

Depression, suicidal ideation, and suicide attempts are other significant issues for transgender youth. One study of suicidal behaviors and their correlates in transgender youth found that more than half of the FTM subjects had sometimes or often had serious thoughts of taking their lives, and 33% had actually made a suicide attempt.[28] In trying to clarify what differences might exist between transgender youth who made suicide attempts and those who did not, this same study looked at childhood gender nonconformity, childhood parental abuse, and body esteem. Suicide attempts were not correlated with childhood gender nonconformity. There was, however, a correlation between parental physical and verbal abuse and suicide attempts, as well as correlations between negative feelings about the body (specifically related to weight and how the youth thought his body was regarded by peers) and suicide attempts.[28]

A recent study from The Netherlands found that when adolescents and adults at their gender clinic were compared on measures of psychological health, the adolescents actually seemed to be better than the adults.[29] The authors speculated that because these youth were getting assistance with gender role change earlier through puberty suppression or hormone therapy, they may have felt more supported and experienced less harm associated with stigmatization than did the adults.

TREATMENT OPTIONS

If the adolescent does have significant gender dysphoria, a variety of treatment options are available. Ways in which a mental health professional may be of assistance to an adolescent and his or her family after the initial assessment are numerous. There is a role for education for parents and the transgender adolescent; this must include education for parents and adolescents regarding the diagnosis of GID/gender dysphoria. The recommendations of the World Professional Association for Transgender Health's Standards of Care[30] regarding the evaluation, treatment, and follow-up for those interested in sex reassignment surgery need to be discussed. Careful evaluation of the diagnosis and following strict criteria for transitioning have been found essential by the Dutch group.[31,32] Parents and teens need to hear realistic descriptions of what hormones and surgery can and cannot do for a person seeking sex reassignment surgery. The important role that parents and other family members can play in understanding, supporting, and advocating for their adolescent must be stressed. When the young person still has a good deal of ambivalence or lack of clarity about gender identity, individual therapy for the adolescent is highly recommended. A therapist can help the adolescent decide on the best adaptation, or can provide support during the "real-life experience"[30] of living, attending school, or working as a boy. If the adolescent is confident about his/her gender identity and the path s/he wishes to take, but the family is opposed, then family therapy will be an important adjunct.

Adolescents in the past have had to wait until the age of 18 years to be eligible for hormonal or surgical interventions. They were not considered to be mature enough to know what would be best for them. The awareness of how detrimental it has been for some adolescents to be forced to wait while the physical changes of puberty progressed unabated has led to changes in this policy, as the means to suspend puberty have become more widely available. In very recent years, endocrinologists and mental health clinicians have been willing to consider puberty suppression or suspension for early adolescents and cross-sex hormone therapy once adolescents reach the age of 16[33–36]; indeed, the Endocrine Society has advocated for such treatment of transgender adolescents.[37] The clinician who has evaluated and treated the patient is the one who will be responsible for writing a letter stating that this adolescent is ready and would benefit from puberty suspension, hormone therapy, or surgery (the latter at age $\geq$18 years). It is considered best practice to follow the Standards of Care[30] and cite this in such a referral letters.

Community resources for transgender youth and their families vary depending on the geographic location. Some cities have support groups for trans youth already in place; others do not. Online resources are available and especially important for FTM youth who may not have access to support groups, or for parents wanting further information or support in coming to terms with their child's gender variance. A list of online resources may be found in **Box 1**. These are resources that families may benefit from utilizing in addition to youth. Examples of such resources are: TransYouth Family Allies and Parents, Families and Friends of Lesbians and Gays (PFLAG).

Box 1
Online community resources

About.com. Gay, Lesbian, Bisexual and Transgender Resources: http://gayteens.about.com/od/transgenderteenissues/Transgender_Teen_Issues.htm

Advocates for Youth. I Think I Might Be Transgender, Now What Do I Do?: http://www.advocatesforyouth.org/storage/advfy/documents/transgender.pdf

Hudson's FTM Resource Guide: http://www.ftmguide.org/

Lambda Legal. Bending the Mold: An Action Kit for Transgender Students: http://data.lambdalegal.org/publications/downloads/btm_bending-the-mold.pdf

TNET: PFLAG's Transgender Network. PFLAG: Parents, Families and Friends of Lesbians and Gays: http://www.pflag.org/

TransYouthFamily Allies: http://www.imatyfa.org/

It is also evident that educational programs are needed for mental health professionals so they can be more knowledgeable and competent in the assessment and treatment of gender dysphoric youth and their families.[28] Although there is a need for specialty gender clinics, they may not always be available or easily accessible. Therefore, child and adolescent psychiatrists in the community can be of great assistance in completing a thorough psychiatric evaluation and providing follow-up care to assist transgender youth and their families.

REFERENCES

1. American Psychiatric Association (APA). Diagnostic and statistical manual of mental disorders. 4th edition. Text Revised. Washington (DC): Author; 2000.
2. Devor H. FTM: female-to-male transsexuals in society. Bloomington: Indiana University Press; 1997.
3. Lee T. Trans(re)lations: lesbian and female to male transsexual accounts of identity. Womens Stud Int Forum 2001;24:347–57.
4. Pazos S. Practice with female-to-male transgendered youth. J Gay Lesbian Soc Serv 1999;10:65–82.
5. Wallien MSC, Cohen-Kettenis PT. Psychosexual outcome of gender-dysphoric children. J Am Acad Child Adolesc Psychiatry 2008;47:1413–23.
6. Drummond KD, Bradley SJ, Peterson-Badali M, et al. A follow-up study of girls with gender identity disorder. Dev Psychol 2008;44:34–45.
7. Zucker KJ. Gender identity development and issues. Child Adolesc Psychiatric Clin N Am 2004;13:551–68.
8. Steensma TD, Biemond R, de Boer F, et al. Desisting and persisting gender dysphoria after childhood: a qualitative follow-up study. Clin Child Psychology Psychiatry 2011 Jan 7 [Epub ahead of print].
9. Kenagy GP, Hsieh C-M. The risk less known: female-to-male transgender persons' vulnerability to HIV infection. AIDS Care 2005;17:195–207.
10. Diamond LM, Butterworth M. Questioning gender and sexual identity: dynamic links over time. Sex Roles 2008;59:365–76.
11. Devor AH. Witnessing and mirroring: a 14-stage model of transsexual identity formation. Journal of Gay and Lesbian Psychotherapy 2004;8:41–67.
12. Bockting W, Coleman E. Developmental stages of the transgender coming-out process: toward an integrated identity. In: Ettner R, Monstrey S, Eyler AE, editors. Principles of transgender medicine and surgery. Binghamton (NY): Haworth Press; 2007. p. 185–208.
13. Holman CW, Goldberg J. Ethical, legal, and psychosocial issues in care of transgender adolescents. International Journal of Transgenderism 2006;9:95–110.
14. Newman LK. Sex, gender and culture: issues in the definition, assessment and treatment of gender identity disorder. Clin Child Psychol Psychiatr 2002;7:352–9.
15. Olson J, Forbes C, Belzer M. Management of the transgender adolescent. Arch Pediatr Adolesc Med 2011;165:171–6.
16. Deogracias JJ, Johnson LL, Meyer-Bahlburg HFL, et al. The gender identity/gender dysphoria questionnaire for adolescents and adults. J Sex Res 2007;44:370–9.
17. Wallien MSC, Veenstra R, Kreukels BPC, et al. Peer group status of gender dysphoric children: a sociometric study. Arch Sex Behav 2010;39:553–60.
18. Devor H. FTM: female-to-male transsexuals in society. Bloomington: Indiana University Press; 1997.
19. Morgan SW, Stevens PE. Transgender identity development as represented by a group of female-to-male transgendered adults. Issues Ment Health Nurs 2008;29:585–99.

20. Rubin H. Self-made men: identity and embodiment among transsexual men. Nashville: Vanderbilt University Press; 2003.
21. Wallien MSC, Swaab H, Cohen-Kettenis PT. Psychiatric comorbidity among children with gender identity disorder. J Am Acad Child Adolesc Psychiatry 2007;46:1307–14.
22. Achenbach TM. Integrative guide to the 1991 CBCL/4-18, YSR, and TRF profiles. Burlington: University of Vermont; 1991.
23. Cohen-Kettenis PT, Owen A, Kaijser V, et al. Demographic characteristics, social competence, and behavior problems in children with gender identity disorder: a cross-national, cross-clinic comparative analysis. J Abn Child Psychol 2003;31: 41–53.
24. Peirce B. Boy's don't cry. Los Angeles: Fox Searchlight Pictures; 1999.
25. Muska S, Olafsdóttir G. The Brandon Teena story. New York: Zeitgeist Films; 1998.
26. Scholinski D. The last time I wore a dress. New York: Riverhead Press; 1997.
27. Denizet-Lewis B. About a boy who isn't. New York Times Magazine; May 26, 2002. Available at: www.nytimes.com. Accessed May 15, 2011.
28. Grossman AH, D'Augelli AR. Transgender youth and life-threatening behaviors. Suicide Life Threat Behav 2007;37:527–37.
29. deVries ALC, Kreukels BPC, Steensma TD, et al. Comparing adult and adolescent transsexuals: An MMPI-2 and MMPI—a study. Psychiatry Res 2011;186:414–8.
30. World Professional Association for Transgender Health (WPATH). The Harry Benjamin International Gender Dysphoria Association's standards of care for gender identity disorders, Sixth Version. Available at: http://www.wpath.org/publications_standards.cfm.
31. Cohen-Kettenis PT, Van Goozen SHM. Sex reassignment of adolescent transsexuals: a follow-up study. J Am Acad Child Adolesc Psychiatry 1997;36:263–71.
32. Smith YLS, Van Goozen SHM, Cohen-Kettenis PT. Adolescents with gender identity disorder who were accepted or rejected for sex reassignment surgery: a prospective follow-up study. J Am Acad Child Adolesc Psychiatry 2001;40:472–81.
33. Delemarre-van der Waal H, Cohen-Kettenis P. Clinical management of gender identity disorder in adolescents: a protocol on psychological and paediatric endocrinology aspects. Eur J Endocrinol 2006;155:S131–7.
34. Cohen-Kettenis PT, Delemarre-van der Waal H, Gooren LJG. The treatment of adolescent transsexuals: changing insights. J Sex Med 2008;5:1892–7.
35. Gibson B. Care of the child with the desire to change genders—part II: Female-to-male transition. Pediatric Nurs 2010;36:112–7.
36. Gooren LJG, Delemarre-van de Waal H. The feasibility of endocrine interventions in juvenile transsexuals. J Psychol Human Sex 1996;8:69–74.
37. Hembree WC, Cohen-Kettenis PT, Delemarre-van de Waal HA, et al. Endocrine treatment of transsexual persons: an Endocrine Society clinical practice guideline. J Clin Endocrinol Metab 2009;94:3132–54.

Treatment of Adolescents With Gender Dysphoria in the Netherlands

Peggy T. Cohen-Kettenis, PhD[a],*, Thomas D. Steensma, MSc[a],
Annelou L.C. de Vries, MD, PhD[b]

KEYWORDS

- Gender dysphoria • Puberty suppression
- Gender identity disorder
- Gonadotropin-releasing hormone analogues • Adolescents

Adolescents with gender dysphoria seek help for a variety of problems. Some have intense distress about the incongruence between their natal sex and gender identity and expect that clinicians will provide them with hormones and gender reassignment (GR) surgery as quickly as possible. Others feel only some unease with or confusion about their gender identity and try to find ways to live with these feelings. The gender dysphoria may have started long before puberty or be recent. It might have been a response to certain experiences or have been present without a clear starting point. There are also huge differences between adolescents in their ability to handle the complexities and adversities that often accompany gender variance. The ways in which the environment has responded to their gender variant behavior can vary from accepting and supporting to rejecting and stigmatizing. When these adolescents present at clinics, they may have a broad range of coexisting psychiatric problems. In recent years, many of these youth have come to gender identity clinics with a straight focus on GR (ie, cross-sex hormone treatment and surgery). However, not only in adult gender identity clinics but also in clinics treating adolescents, nonclassic presentations increasingly need a diagnosis and some form of treatment.[1]

In 1987, the first gender identity clinic for children and adolescents was opened in the Netherlands at what is now called the Center of Expertise on Gender Dysphoria. Since then more than 800 children and adolescents have attended the gender identity clinic. Meanwhile, ideas about treatment have greatly changed. Diagnostic protocols and instruments for adolescents have been developed, and medical interventions,

The authors have nothing to disclose.
[a] Department of Medical Psychology and Medical Social Work, VU University Medical Center, PO Box 7057, 1007 MB Amsterdam, the Netherlands
[b] Department of Child and Adolescent Psychiatry, VU University Medical Center, PO Box 7057, 1007 MB Amsterdam, the Netherlands
* Corresponding author.
E-mail address: PT.Cohen-Kettenis@vumc.nl

including the halting of puberty, have become available for gender dysphoric adolescents.[2-4] Various professional organizations and clinics have published treatment guidelines.[5-8] The introduction of gonadotropin-releasing hormone (GnRH) analogues to suppress puberty especially signified an important change in the clinical management of gender dysphoria in youth. However, puberty suppression is not without criticism.[9]

Because the gender identity clinic in the Netherlands took a leading role in developing this model of care, the model is sometimes called the "Dutch approach."[10] In this article the authors describe diagnosis and treatment as they have developed it at their clinic. The authors use *Diagnostic and Statistical Manual of Mental Disorders, Fourth Edition, Text Revision* (DSM-IV-TR)[11] nomenclature and criteria, although they are aware of the upcoming changes that are likely to be introduced in the DSM-5.

DEVELOPMENTAL TRAJECTORIES

Gender-variant behavior and even the desire to be of an other gender can be either a phase or a variation of normal development without any adverse consequences for a child's current functioning (eg, Bartlett and colleagues[12]). Prospective studies showed that the presence of childhood gender variance in clinical populations is associated with later homosexuality or bisexuality, as well as gender dysphoria, in adulthood.[13-22] Nevertheless, even in clinical populations, in over about 25% of cases the gender dysphoria does not persist from childhood into adulthood.

In contrast to childhood gender dysphoria, during adolescence it seems much more unlikely that gender dysphoria will desist. Adolescents who were gender dysphoric in childhood and present at gender identity clinics soon after puberty rarely refrain from GR later in adolescence.[2,23] In a study by de Vries and colleagues,[24] adolescents who started puberty suppression at an average age of 14.75 years to enable exploration of their gender dysphoria and treatment wish were still gender dysphoric nearly 2 years later, and all chose to start cross-sex hormone treatment, the first step of actual GR, at a mean age of 16.64 years.

THE DUTCH APPROACH

The recommended procedure in the Standards of Care of the World Professional Association for Transgender Health (WPATH; www.wpath.org), an international professional organization in the field of gender dysphoria and transsexualism, is to come to a GR decision in various phases.[8] In the first phase, someone has to fulfill DSM or International Classification of Diseases criteria for gender identity disorder (GID) or transsexualism.[11,25] The next phase consists of real-life experience, and hormones of the desired gender are prescribed. The last phase consists of various types of surgery to change the genitals and other sex characteristics. The Amsterdam clinic has always largely followed this procedure.

The Diagnostic Procedure

Creating a working relationship

When working with gender dysphoric adolescents, it is important to create a working relationship. It helps to explain that clinicians are neutral regarding the outcome of the diagnostic process. If GR seems to be the best solution to the apparent gender issues, medical interventions, including puberty suppression, are available. If other solutions seem to be better, other types of interventions are advised. This attitude is most helpful in allowing the youth to openly explore gender dysphoric feelings and treatment wishes.

Obtaining information
In the diagnostic phase, the gender identity problem and potential related problems are examined comprehensively by the mental health clinician, who is usually a clinical child psychologist. Eligibility and readiness for puberty suppression and GR are considered during this phase. Some youth wish that there were medical tests to objectively measure gender dysphoria, but clearly these do not exist. Yet it is extremely important not to refer the wrong individuals for medical interventions. Mental health professionals are largely dependent on the information given by the adolescents and their parents to assess treatment eligibility. Adolescents and parents are usually seen together at the first session, which enables the mental health professional to interview them jointly and separately and observe any relevant family interactions. During the intake and subsequent sessions, most of which are with the adolescent, information is obtained on various aspects of the general and psycho-sexual development of the adolescent. Before visiting the gender identity clinic, parents fill out a number of instruments such as the Child Behavior Checklist (CBCL)[26] and a self-developed questionnaire on the adolescent's development. The CBCL Youth Self Report is administered to the adolescent.[27]

Information is also obtained about current cross-gender feelings and behavior, current school functioning, peer relations, and family functioning. With regard to sexuality, sexual experiences, sexual attractions, sexual relationships, the subjective meaning of cross-dressing, sexual fantasies accompanying cross-dressing (if any), and body image are explored.

A psychodiagnostic assessment not only measures gender-related issues such as gender dysphoria and body satisfaction (see Zucker[4] for an overview of instruments), but also general aspects of psychological functioning: intellectual abilities, coping abilities, psychopathology, and self-esteem.

The assessment of the relationships within the family and family functioning are less standardized than the other aspects of the diagnostic procedure. Yet this assessment provides important information because parents (or other caregivers) are the ones the adolescent has to rely on during the period in adolescence that medical interventions are provided. This period can take more than 6 years when the diagnostic phase is started at the age of 12 years. Clinicians therefore have regular contact with the family during the diagnostic and GR process.

Giving information
In order to create realistic expectations with regard to the adolescents' future lives, the clinician gives information on the possibilities and limitations of GR and other types of treatment such as psychological interventions. Clinicians also discuss the broader impact of GR. The loss of fertility is one important aspect. Although a rare event, older natal male adolescents who are already beyond the first pubertal (Tanner) stages when assessed at the clinic may choose to freeze their sperm. Younger adolescents usually do not want to wait until Tanner stages 4 or 5 but prefer to start with puberty-suppressing hormones before they are fertile. Much of the information is given early in the procedure because some may refrain from GR as soon as they realize what GR actually entails. Clinicians further explore with the youth whether the gender dysphoria might be solved by either psychological interventions or hormone or surgical interventions only rather than a complete GR.

Like in other countries, in the Netherlands being overweight or obese is becoming more and more prevalent.[28] This trend is also observable in gender dysphoric youth applying for GR. Another health issue concerns cigarette smoking. In 2010, about 20% of Dutch youth between 10 and 20 years reported to have smoked in the last 4 weeks.[29] As the pediatric endocrinologists and plastic surgeons consider obesity and smoking as factors that seriously impact effects of hormone treatment and surgical outcome, attention is increasingly given to these lifestyle issues. Adolescents are encouraged to work on their eating and smoking habits long before the actual treatment starts. This is done not only by the diagnostician. If an adolescent is likely to be referred for medical interventions, he or she will visit the pediatric endocrinologist for an advisory consultation. The authors have chosen for this procedure in order to properly inform the youth and their parents about the medical aspects of the treatment. At this time the adolescent also has a medical screening (see also Hembree and colleagues[7]).

Informing the adolescent about the various consequences of GR concerns so many topics and touches upon such complex issues that it is impossible to do so in one session. The issues are discussed throughout the diagnostic procedure in order to allow for a truly informed consent, but some are also discussed in later phases of the GR process.

Child psychiatric assessment

Shortly before the final advice on eligibility and readiness for medical interventions is discussed in the child and adolescent gender team, a child psychiatric consultation is performed. The child psychiatrist is also a part of the team. This involvement ensures that there are always two mental health clinicians who know the adolescent and the family and that the decision to start treatment is not taken on the basis of personal contacts with only one team member. In addition, because a substantial number of the referred adolescents have psychiatric comorbidity with almost 10% having autistic spectrum disorders (ASD), a psychiatric evaluation is important to address these problems.[30,31]

Team decision

An advisory consultation concludes the diagnostic procedure. If the recommendation is to start puberty suppression, this decision is always made by the whole team after a discussion of the case. It seems that about one-quarter of the adolescent referrals at the Amsterdam clinic do not fulfill diagnostic criteria for GID. Most of the adolescents drop out early in the diagnostic procedure for this reason or because other problems are prominent.[24]

Treatment: Psychological Interventions

Indications for psychological interventions

When the gender identity problem requires further exploration, psychological and/or family problems exist, or psychiatric comorbidity occurs, some form of psychological treatment is offered or sought close to the youth's home. This advice is also given to adolescents with GID to whom medical interventions (most likely puberty suppression) will be provided, especially in vulnerable youngsters. Problems that may require either psychological interventions only, or before or in combination with medical interventions, are as follows:

- *Gender confusion.* Referred adolescents are sometimes only uncertain about their gender. For example, young male homosexuals may have a history of stereotypical feminine interests and dressing in girls' clothes. They sometimes mistake their homosexuality for a GID (see Tuerk article elsewhere in this issue) despite decreased cross-gender interests and activities after puberty and a disappearance of the gender dysphoric feelings. A lack of acceptance of their homosexuality may make them consider GR a solution to their problem. Other adolescent males fulfilling the DSM-IV-TR criteria for transvestic fetishism interpret their desire to wear female clothing, with or without accompanying sexual arousal, as a sign of GID and need for GR. Especially for adolescents, it is difficult to know whether this is a permanent situation or just an experimental phase in someone who will never seek GR.

- *Aversion toward sexuality or sexed body parts.* In (relatively rare) cases, a wish for genital ablation exists in persons who prefer to be sexless but have no cross-gender identity. This desire has been described as the Skoptic syndrome[32] or as male-to-eunuch identity disorder in males who seek castration voluntarily without wanting to acquire the female characteristics (eg, Johnson[33]). It is likely that the taboo that still exists on this phenomenon makes adolescents reluctant to present with such a treatment wish at the authors' clinic.

- *GID without GR.* Gender dysphoric adolescents who do not desire complete GR (both cross-sex hormones and surgery) may try to integrate masculine and feminine aspects of the self and adopt an androgynous, bigendered, or "genderqueer" form of expression. Again, such a treatment wish is relatively rare in adolescents who present at the authors' clinic. It is conceivable that suffering from GID without having a desire for GR signifies a the result of developmental route that takes more time to be completed.

- *Psychiatric comorbidities.* Comorbid psychiatric problems need to be addressed to ensure that the diagnostic or treatment process is not unduly disturbed. When comorbidities are addressed, adolescents can be eligible for puberty suppression. To achieve an uneventful treatment, good, regular contact with the local mental health clinicians is necessary.[30] If the observed problems are destabilizing and there is an insufficient guarantee that the youth has a commitment to the relationship with the psychologist and medical doctors, which is necessary for this type of a physical interventions, medical treatment is postponed until the adolescent or his or her situation has become sufficiently stable. In the authors' clinic, treatment seemed to be delayed more frequently in youths who suffered from psychiatric comorbidity, were less likely to live with both biological parents, and had a lower intelligence. On average, adolescents with psychiatric comorbidities were older at the time of referral.[30]

- *ASD-related diagnostic difficulties.* Youth with ASD often present themselves at gender identity clinics. As has been described by de Vries and colleagues,[31] the conviction to have a cross-gender identity may exist parallel to the ASD but may also be part of the rigid convictions that belong to autism. It is a challenge to disentangle the gender and ASD components. When adolescents with ASD are considered eligible for medical intervention including puberty suppression, treatment has to be introduced very carefully, and each step must take place in close consultation with the other mental health clinicians involved in the treatment or counseling of the adolescent.[31]

Types of psychological interventions

The range of treatment goals is broad, because many factors may underlie the issues gender dysphoric youths are struggling with (see also de Vries and colleagues[5,34]). These youth may be directed toward dealing with the gender identity issue itself, for instance if there is uncertainty about the experienced gender identity or hesitance about the type of medical interventions that may solve the discrepancy between experienced gender and natal sex. Interventions sometimes focus on the consequences of one's gender variance.

Adolescents may struggle with shame about being different, guilt toward parents, or low self-esteem. In some cases they suffer from social repercussions of being gender-variant, such as exclusion from certain social circles or being teased, bullied, ridiculed, or harassed.[35,36] Psychotherapy can help these adolescents to become more self-confident, not be bothered by unnecessary feelings of shame and guilt, and/or enhance social skills.

Although the authors usually offer individuals who want to explore their options for coping with gender dysphoria some form of individual therapy, having contact with other transgender youngsters is helpful too. Observing other adolescents dealing with their gender identity concerns, sharing information, and peer support is often experienced as highly beneficial. In the Netherlands, adolescents can join meetings for gender dysphoric adolescents. These meetings are organized by a support group such as Transvisie. These meetings do not have a therapeutic goal but are intended to offer a safe and informal social setting to meet peers. The consequences of such contacts, however, can be very therapeutic.

Psychotherapy offered to gender dysphoric adolescents who are considering GR is supportive of GR. This means the adolescent is made aware that any outcome of the therapy (whether it is acceptance of living in the social role congruent with the natal sex, partial treatment, or complete GR) is acceptable as long as it leads to the relief of the adolescent's gender dysphoria and a better quality of life.

For adolescents who start GR, various topics have to be brought up repeatedly because their views and experiences often change over time. Examples are relationships with peers, sexuality, and infertility. One discusses aspects of sexuality with a 13-year-old, who is only fantasizing about falling in love, differently than with an 18-year-old, who tries to find ways of having sex while having a body that is not yet completely congruent with the experienced gender. Youth will profit most from having a balanced view of the short-term and long-term costs and benefits of GR, and this balance is what they may learn in psychotherapy or counseling sessions. Communicating, dating, or initiating contact with potential romantic partners can be hampered by certain characteristics of the person such as extreme shyness, lack of self-confidence, or perfectionism. Such characteristics need specific attention to facilitate future partnerships. Like other adolescents, gender dysphoric adolescents need adequate information about sexuality in general. For some it is necessary to point out the chances of aggressive reactions when they engage in sexual encounters, in case the sexual partner is not aware of the adolescent's natal sex.

Even if secondary sex characteristics have hardly developed because of timely puberty suppression and an early social role change, some adolescents feel frustrated because in their opinion they have to wait too long for their estrogen or androgen treatment to feminize/masculinize in the same ways as their age peers. When they have started cross-sex hormone treatment, waiting for surgery can be equally frustrating and if not addressed can lead to social withdrawal.

Sometimes family therapy is necessary to help resolve conflicts between family members. For example, parents may have different views about how to handle their child, or the adolescent may want to express gender in ways that other family members are not comfortable with. Also, parents and/or adolescents can have trouble distinguishing between what is related to the gender dysphoria and what is not. In the counseling of families, parents are supported in determining realistic demands and in working on the development of healthy boundaries and limits.

The authors also consider regular contact with a mental health practitioner at their clinic necessary for adequate preparation for the next treatment steps. For instance, adolescents have to be aware of medical risks that arise with an unhealthy lifestyle, and trans girls' (natal boys with a female gender identity) need laser hair removal on a portion of the scrotal area (something they often do not like to do) when preparing for vaginoplasty. The adolescents should also be conscious of the practical consequences of medical interventions. For instance, they will need to take hormones for the rest of their life, and trans girls will need to dilate their neovagina after surgery if they are not sexually active. When surgery is discussed, unrealistic expectations about the depth of the neovagina or size of the neophallus have to be put into perspective.

For those who do not easily verbalize their feelings, psychomotor therapy can be helpful to let adolescents feel more at ease with their body and to learn to talk more easily about their concerns.

Treatment: Medical Interventions

Puberty suppression

Eligibility for puberty suppression. If adolescents do have a diagnosis of GID, they may be eligible for puberty suppression by means of GnRH analogues. The authors believe that offering this medical intervention minimizes the harm to the youth while maximizing the opportunity for a good quality of life including social and sexual relationships, and that it respects the wishes of the person involved.[37]

GnRH analogues put a halt to the development of secondary sex characteristics. Originally GnRH analogues were used in the treatment of precocious puberty. Because gonadal function is reactivated soon after cessation of treatment,[38] GnRH analogue treatment can be considered as "buying time" rather than actual treatment.

Current eligibility criteria for puberty suppression are an early history of GID that has intensified rather than decreased during the early pubertal phases, no serious psychosocial problems interfering with the diagnostic assessment or treatment, and a good comprehension of the impact of GR on one's life. It is also considered important that there is enough support from the family or other caregivers. The adolescent should have reached Tanner stage 2 to 3 and be older than 12 years of age.[3,39] Starting around Tanner stages 2 to 3, the very first physical changes are still reversible.[3] Some experience with one's physical puberty is required because the authors assume that experiencing one's own puberty is diagnostically useful. It is at the onset of puberty that it becomes clear whether the gender dysphoria will desist or persist.[40] Besides, some cognitive and emotional maturation is desirable when starting these physical medical interventions. In addition, Dutch adolescents are legally competent to make a medical decision together with their parents' consent, at age 12. The age criterion of 12 years, however, is under discussion, because many natal girls are already beyond Tanner stage 3 when they are 12 years old. It is conceivable that when more information about the safety of early hormone treatment becomes available, the age limit will be further adjusted (de Vries AL, Steensma TD, Wagenaar EC, and colleagues, unpublished data, 2011).

Puberty suppression. If the eligibility criteria are met, GnRH analogues are used to suppress puberty (eg, triptorelin, 3.75 mg every 4 weeks).[7,39] An extra dose is given after 2 weeks of GnRH analogue treatment to counteract the initial surge of sex hormones. Because the effects are reversible, this treatment phase could be considered an extended diagnostic phase. Knowing that the treatment will put a halt to the physical puberty development often results in a vast reduction of the distress that the physical feminization of masculinization was producing. Also, the early suppression of the development of secondary sex characteristics makes passing in the desired gender role easier than when treatment is delayed until adulthood. This early suppression entails a great advantage for passing in the desired role throughout one's life. Clinicians, however, explain to the adolescent and family that puberty suppression does not automatically imply that cross-sex hormone treatment will take place later on. To make a well-informed and balanced decision, adolescents see their psychologist or psychiatrist regularly in the years that they are on GnRH analogues. These sessions are meant to evaluate feelings about a transition on a permanent basis, with increasing knowledge of what a future life in the desired gender role might look like. The adolescents are also regularly given consideration in a weekly multidisciplinary conference in which the pediatric endocrinologist also participates. As soon as necessary, extra help is deployed or the trajectory is adjusted.

If youth suffer from psychiatric problems but the mental health treatment they receive is adequate to ensure that the diagnostic or treatment process is not unduly disturbed, they are still eligible for puberty suppression.

Transitioning. Puberty suppression gives adolescents time to quietly explore their gender identity and GR wish, even without informing the wider environment that they are contemplating GR. However, most gender dysphoric youths choose to live in the desired gender role simultaneously with the beginning of puberty suppression. The adolescents and their family are supported in this process by the clinicians to allow for a smooth process. Many youths also obtain help from the aforementioned support group, Transvisie. The group has volunteers who may assist the youth, parents, or school during the process. It is, however, not a requirement to transition socially as long as cross-sex hormones are not taken.

Cross-sex hormone treatment

Eligibility for cross-sex hormone treatment. In the Dutch protocol, gender dysphoric adolescents are eligible for the first step of the actual GR when they have reached the age of 16. This has been chosen because in the Netherlands (as well as in many other countries) young people are then considered able to make independent medical decisions. Whereas parental approval is not officially required, the Amsterdam clinic prefers their consent, because most adolescents are still very much dependent on their caretakers. Besides, by the age of 16, adolescents have to meet the same criteria as for puberty suppression (except for the Tanner stage criterion). Although most of the youths will have already made a social transition, it is an absolute requirement that they will make the social gender role change as soon as the cross-hormones are taken. This requirement is because soon after the start of treatment, sex characteristics of the desired gender will become visible to others.

Cross-sex hormone treatment. If an adolescent still wants to start the actual GR at 16 years, feminizing puberty is induced in natal boys by prescribing 5 μg/kg 17β estradiol per day and increasing the dose every 6 months by 5 μg/kg. An adult dose of 2 mg per day is given when the patient reaches 18 years of age. In natal girls, male puberty is induced with testosterone esters starting at 25 mg/m^2 per 2 weeks intramuscularly. The dose is increased every 6 months by 25 mg/m^2. At age 18 years an adult dose is given of 250 mg per 3 to 4 weeks. In trans girls the estrogens will result in breast growth and a female fat distribution. In trans boys the androgens will result in a more muscular development, particularly in the upper body; a lower, male-sounding voice; facial and body hair growth; and clitoris growth.[3,7]

At some point the operations are close at hand. As noted previously, the possibilities and limitations of the surgery (eg, various types of metaidoioplasty or phalloplasty, or no genital surgery for trans boys) about which the adolescent will have to make choices need to be discussed more extensively.[41]

Surgery
Eligibility for surgery. When adolescents in the authors' clinic reach 18 years of age, as previous phases have consolidated the diagnosis and social transition has been successful, they are eligible for the next treatment step, the GR surgeries. Trans boys may undergo several operations: if they came relatively late to the clinic and already had some breast development, mastectomy; hysterectomy/ovariectomy; colpectomy (also called vaginectomy); and, if desired, operations on the external genitalia (metaidoioplasty or phalloplasty). Trans girls usually undergo partial penectomy with vaginoplasty and, if necessary, at their own financial expense, breast augmentation. Trans girls who began puberty suppression at an early age often have insufficient penile skin for a classic vaginoplasty and need an adjusted surgical procedure, such as a technique using colon tissue.

Dilemmas
The treatment of young gender dysphoric adolescents has received a variety of criticisms (eg, by Korte and colleagues,[9] Meyenburg,[42] and Viner and colleagues[43]). Some state that a diagnosis of GID cannot be made in adolescence because in this developmental phase gender identity is still fluctuating. Others fear that puberty suppression will inhibit a spontaneous formation of a gender identity corresponding with one's natal sex. In the authors' clinic population, however, GID seems to be highly persistent from early puberty on, and certainly after Tanner stage 2 or 3. None of the younger and older adolescents diagnosed with GID and considered eligible for GR dropped out of treatment during the GR procedure or regretted GR.[44–46]

Other concerns relate to bone density, body height, and brain development. Peak bone mass may not be achieved and/or there might be body segment disproportion. The first data of a Dutch cohort of adolescents who had been treated with GnRH analogues suggest that after an initial slowing in bone maturation it significantly caught up after the commencement of cross-sex steroid hormone treatment[3,47] (Schagen SE, Cohen-Kettenis PT, van Coeverden-van den Heijkant SC, and colleagues, unpublished data, 2011). Body proportions, as measured by sitting height and sitting-height/height ratio, remained in the normal range. Early treatment may result in a final height in the normal natal female range for trans girls. For trans boys, a timely administration of oxandrolone, a synthetic anabolic steroid that influences height development, may result in acceptable natal male height. Although the effects of puberty suppression on brain development have not been systematically studied, clinically there seems to be no effect on social, emotional, and school functioning.

Not treating gender dysphoric adolescents is not a neutral option. Delaying treatment until adulthood or even until older adolescence may have its psychological drawbacks. Some youth develop psychiatric problems such as depression and suicidality, anxiety, or oppositional defiant disorders, or they may become school dropouts or react with complete social withdrawal. Puberty suppression seems to quickly result in a relief of their distress and a significant improvement in their quality of life. When gender dysphoric youth are denied access to GR, they might seek medication illegally or respond to their distress in other irresponsible ways.

If treated early in puberty, these youth may also be spared the burden of having to live with irreversible signs of the "wrong" secondary sex characteristics (eg, scarring because of breast removal in trans boys; having a male voice and male facial and bodily features in trans girls). Having no or only few visible sex characteristics of one's natal sex obviously is an enormous and lifelong advantage. Furthermore, early treatment will likely make certain forms of surgery redundant or less invasive (eg, breast reduction in trans boys). It is not surprising that follow-up studies among adult transsexuals show that unfavorable postoperative outcome seems to be related to a later rather than an early start of GR (for reviews, see Cohen-Kettenis and Gooren,[48] Pfäfflin and Junge,[49] and Ross and Need[50]).

SUMMARY

Puberty suppression in young gender dysphoric adolescents seems to be beneficial and able to prevent harmful effects of growing up with a body that is incongruent with one's gender identity. Despite the reservations that many clinicians had when this protocol was introduced, views on this approach are rapidly changing.[39,51] In the last 5 years a fair number of clinics in and outside Europe (eg, in Belgium, Germany, Finland, Italy, Norway, Spain, Switzerland, Australia, and the United States) have adopted an identical clinical approach. The first studies showing promising effects (de Vries AL, Steensma TD, Wagenaar EC, and colleagues, unpublished data 2011)[24,44,45] and the increasing numbers of gender dysphoric youth who apply for medical interventions are probably related to these policy changes.

However, research on the effects of GR, starting with GnRH analogues treatment, is still scarce, and understandable concerns about potential harm have to be taken seriously. The initial studies need to be expanded in scope and corroborated by results from other centers to ensure that the treatment is safe enough. It would also be useful to compare other treatment protocols with the one described in this article.

REFERENCES

1. Bockting WO. Psychotherapy and the real-life experience: from gender dichotomy to gender diversity. Sexologies 2008;17:211–24.
2. Cohen-Kettenis PT, Pfäfflin F. Transgenderism and intersexuality in childhood and adolescence. Thousand Oaks (CA): SAGE Publications; 2003.
3. Delemarre-van de Waal HA, Cohen-Kettenis PT. Clinical management of gender identity disorder in adolescents: a protocol on psychological and paediatric endocrinology aspects. Eur J Endocrinology 2006;155:131–7.
4. Zucker KJ. Measurement of psychosexual differentiation. Arch Sex Behav 2005;34: 375–88.
5. de Vries AL, Cohen-Kettenis PT, Delemarre-van de Waal HA. Clinical management of gender dysphoria in adolescents. International Journal of Transgenderism 2007;9:83–94.
6. Di Ceglie, D, Sturge C, Sutton A. The Royal College of Psychiatrists: gender identity disorders in children and adolescents: guidance for management. International Journal of Transgenderism 1998;2.
7. Hembree, WC, Cohen-Kettenis PT, Delemarre-van de Waal HA, et al. Endocrine treatment of transsexual persons: an endocrine society clinical practice guideline. J Clin Endocrinol Metab 2009;94:3132–54.
8. Meyer W, Bockting WO, Cohen-Kettenis PT, et al. Standards of care for gender identity disorders of the Harry Benjamin International Gender Dysphoria Association. 6th edition. World Professional Association for Transgender Health. J Psychol Human Sexuality 2001;13:1--30.
9. Korte, A, Lehmkuhl U, Goecker D, et al. Gender identity disorders in childhood and adolescence: currently debated concepts and treatment strategies. Dtsch Arztebl Int 2008;105:834–41.

10. Dreger A. Gender identity disorder in childhood: inconclusive advice to parents. Hastings Cent Rep 2009;39:26–9.
11. American Psychiatric Association. Diagnostic and Statistical Manual of Mental Disorders. 4th edition. Text revision. Washington, DC: American Psychiatric Association; 2000.
12. Bartlett NH, Vasey PL, Bukowski WM. Is gender identity disorder in children a mental disorder? Sex Roles 2000;43:753–85.
13. Bakwin H. Deviant gender-role behavior in children: relation to homosexuality. Pediatrics 1968;41:620–29.
14. Davenport CW. A follow-up study of 10 feminine boys. Arch Sex Behav 1986;15:511–17.
15. Drummond KD, Bradley SJ, Peterson-Badali M, et al. A follow-up study of girls with gender identity disorder. Dev Psychol 2008;44:34–45.
16. Green R. The "sissy boy syndrome" and the development of homosexuality. New Haven (CT): Yale University Press; 1987.
17. Kosky RJ. Gender-disordered children: does inpatient treatment help? Med J Aust 1987;146:565–69.
18. Lebovitz PS. Feminine behavior in boys: aspects of its outcome. Am J Psychiatry 1972;128:1283–89.
19. Money J, Russo AJ. Homosexual outcome of discordant gender identity/role: longitudinal follow-up. Journal of Pediatric Psychology 1979;4:29–41.
20. Wallien MS, Cohen-Kettenis PT. Psychosexual outcome of gender-dysphoric children. J Am Acad Child Adolesc Psychiatry 2008;47:1413–23.
21. Zucker KJ, Bradley SJ, Lowry Sullivan CB, et al. A gender identity interview for children. J Pers Assess 1993;61:443–56.
22. Zuger B. Early effeminate behavior in boys: outcome and significance for homosexuality. J Nerv Ment Dis 1984;172:90–7.
23. Zucker KJ. Gender identity disorder.In: Wolfe DA, Mash EJ, editors. Behavioral and emotional disorders in adolescents: nature,assessment, and treatment. New York: Guilford Publications; 2006. p. 535–62.
24. de Vries AL, Steensma TD, Doreleijers TA, et al. Puberty suppression in adolescents with gender identity disorder: a prospective follow-up study. J Sex Med 2011;8:2276-83.
25. World Health Organization. International statistical classification of diseases and related health problems. 10th edition. Geneva (Switzerland): World Health Organization; 1993.
26. Achenbach TM, Edelbrock CS. Manual for the Child Behavior Checklist and Revised Child Behavior Profile. Burlington (VT): University of Vermont, Department of Psychiatry; 1983.
27. Achenbach TM. Manual for the Youth Self-Report. Burlington (VT): University of Vermont, Department of Psychiatry; 1991.
28. Fredriks AM, Buuren van S, Wit JM, et al. Body mass index measurements in 1996–7 compared with 1980. Arch Dis Child 2000;82:107–12.
29. Nagelhout GE. Voor een rook vrije toekomst [For a smoke free future]. Den Haag, Netherlands: STIVORO; 2010 [in Dutch]. Available at: http://www.stivoro.nl/Upload/Kerncijfers%20roken%20in%20Nederland%202010.pdf. Accessed September 4, 2011.
30. de Vries AL, Doreleijers TA, Steensma TD, et al. Psychiatric comorbidity in gender dysphoric adolescents. J Child Psychol Psychiatry 2011;Jun 14. [Epub ahead of print.]
31. de Vries AL, Noens IL, Cohen-Kettenis PT, et al. Autism spectrum disorders in gender dysphoric children and adolescents. J Autism Dev Disord 2010;40:930–6.
32. Coleman E, Cesnik J. Skoptic syndrome: the treatment of an obsessional gender dysphoria with lithium carbonate and psychotherapy. Am J Pychother 1990;44:204–17.

33. Johnson TW, Brett MA, Roberts LF, et al. Eunuchs in contemporary society: characterizing men who are voluntarily castrated (part I). J Sex Med 2007;4:930–45.
34. de Vries AL, Cohen-Kettenis PT, Delemarre-van de Waal HA. Caring for transgender adolescents in BC: suggested guidelines. Vancouver Coastal Health. Available at: http://www.vch.ca/transhealth. Accessed September 4, 2011.
35. Russell ST, Ryan C, Toomey RB, et al. Lesbian, gay, bisexual, and transgender adolescent school victimization: implications for young adult health and adjustment. J Sch Health 2011;81:223–30.
36. Burgess C. Internal and external stress factors associated with the identity development of transgendered youth. In: Mallon GP, editor. Social services with transgendered youth. Binghamton (NY): Harrington Park Press; 1999. p. 35–47.
37. Gillam LH, Hewitt JK, Warne GL. Ethical principles for the management of infants with disorders of sex development. Horm Res Paediatr 2010;74:412–18.
38. Mul D, Hughes IA. The use of GnRH agonists in precocious puberty. Eur J Endocrinol 2008;159:3–8.
39. Cohen-Kettenis PT, Delemarre-van de Waal HA, Gooren LJ. The treatment of adolescent transsexuals: changing insights. J Sex Med 2008;5:1892-7.
40. Steensma TD, Biemond R, de Boer F, et al. Desisting and persisting gender dysphoria after childhood: a qualitative follow-up study. Clinic Child Psychol Psychiatry 2011; Jan 7. [Epub ahead of print.]
41. Cohen-Kettenis PT. Gender identity disorders. In: Gillberg C, Harrington R, Steinhausen H-C, editors. A clinician's handbook of child and adolescent psychiatry. New York: Cambridge University Press; 2006. p. 695–725.
42. Meyenburg B. Gender identity disorder in adolescence: outcomes of psychotherapy. Adolescence 1999;34:305–13.
43. Viner RM, Brain C, Carmichael P, et al. Sex on the brain: dilemmas in the endocrine management of children and adolescents with gender identity disorder. Arch Dis Child 2005;90:A78.
44. Cohen-Kettenis PT, van Goozen SH. Sex reassignment of adolescent transsexuals: a follow-up study. J Am Acad Child Adolesc Psychiatry 1997;36:263–71.
45. Smith YL, van Goozen SH, Cohen-Kettenis PT. Adolescents with gender identity disorder who were accepted or rejected for sex reassignment surgery: a prospective follow-up study. J Am Acad Child Adolesc Psychiatry 2001;40:472–81.
46. Smith YL, van Goozen SH, Kuiper AJ, et al. Sex reassignment: outcomes and predictors of treatment for adolescent and adult transsexuals. Psychol Med 2005;35:89–99.
47. Cohen-Kettenis PT, Schagen SE, Steensma TD. et al. Puberty suppression in a gender-dysphoric adolescent: a 22-year follow-up. Arch Sex Behav 2011;40:843–7.
48. Cohen-Kettenis PT, Gooren LJ. Transsexualism: a review of etiology, diagnosis and treatment. J Psychosom Res 1999;46:315–33.
49. Pfäfflin F, Junge A. Nachuntersuchungen nach Geschlechtsumwandlung—Eine kommentierte Literaturübersicht 1961–1991. In: Pfäfflin F, Junge A, editors. Geschlechtsumwandlung—Abhandlungen zur Transsexualität.Stuttgart. New York: Schattauer; 1992 p. 149–457 [in German].
50. Ross MW, Need JA. Effects of adequacy of gender reassignment surgery on psychological adjustment: a follow-up of fourteen male-to-female patients. Arch Sex Behav 1989;18:145–53.
51. Kreukels BP, Cohen-Kettenis PT. Puberty suppression in gender identity disorder: the Amsterdam experience. Nat Rev Endocrinol 2011;7;466–72.

The Development of a Gender Identity Psychosocial Clinic: Treatment Issues, Logistical Considerations, Interdisciplinary Cooperation, and Future Initiatives

Scott F. Leibowitz, MD[a],*, Norman P. Spack, MD[b,c]

KEYWORDS

- Gender identity • Gender dysphoria • Transgender
- Gender variance • Clinic development
- Postgraduate training

With each recent year, public exposure to the issues of gender identity and sexuality has risen due to the print media, television shows, documentaries, movies, and political debates. All too often, the youth and families behind these stories experience stigma, ostracism, and victimization that have led to tragic consequences including substance abuse, depression, suicide, and even homicide. Despite the existence of 105 academic child and adolescent psychiatric training programs participating in the 2010 National Residency Match Program (NRMP),[1] and perhaps several-hundred more community child and adolescent psychiatric treatment centers across the United States, few specialized interdisciplinary treatment programs specifically tend to the complex clinical needs of gender nonconforming and, more specifically,

Disclosure: The authors have nothing to disclose.
[a] Department of Psychiatry, Children's Hospital Boston, Harvard Medical School, 300 Longwood Avenue, Boston, MA 02115, USA
[b] Division of Endocrinology, Children's Hospital Boston, Harvard Medical School, 300 Longwood Avenue, Boston, MA 02115, USA
[c] Gender Management Service, Children's Hospital Boston, Harvard Medical School, 300 Longwood Avenue, Boston, MA 02115, USA
* Corresponding author.
E-mail address: scott.leibowitz@childrens.harvard.edu

Child Adolesc Psychiatric Clin N Am 20 (2011) 701–724
doi:10.1016/j.chc.2011.07.004
1056-4993/11/$ – see front matter © 2011 Elsevier Inc. All rights reserved.

transgender youth. Reputable medical and psychiatric organizations are starting or continuing to develop and publish clinical guidelines for providers (S. Adelson and R.R. Pleak, personal communication, 2011),[2,3] and providers are increasingly more able to find resources designed to improve "gender and sexuality competence" when treating these youth. While the development of guidelines represents a significant attempt to standardize the clinical approach to gender identity and sexuality in child and adolescent mental health, many of the logistical considerations that focus on the development of a specialized clinic or program remain notably absent from those publications. This article will explore the recent development of a new gender identity and sexuality psychosocial treatment clinic by highlighting many of the logistical barriers and complexities while taking into account the previously explored clinical dilemmas and treatment considerations discussed in the literature. While the scope of this volume focuses specifically on gender nonconforming youth, this article often incorporates discussion of sexual minority youth given the developmental relationship that exists between the distinct categories. The development of a specialized interdisciplinary clinic can facilitate the advancement of knowledge in research, education, and community outreach.

DEFINITIONS AND CONVENTIONS

Issues pertaining to gender identity and sexual orientation are often poorly understood, with terms sometimes being used interchangeably by clinicians, parents, teachers, administrators, and youths. This section defines the relevant terms as they are used throughout the rest of this article. "Sex" refers to an individual's biologic or natal genetic makeup as XY or XX and its anatomic expression. "Gender" refers to the perception of a person's sex on the part of society as male or female. "Gender Role" refers to an individual's expression of social norms conventionally regarded as masculine or feminine in dress, speech, and behavior. "Gender identity" refers to a person's personal sense of self as male or female, usually develops by age 3, and remains stable over the lifetime. "Gender nonconforming" refers to variation in gender role from conventional norms and can also be interchangeably referred to as "gender-variant," "gender discordant," or "gender atypical." "Sexual orientation" is the sex to which an individual is erotically attracted and is composed of sexual fantasy, patterns of physiologic arousal, sexual behavior, personal identity, and social role. "Gender dysphoria" is the subjective mood/affect disturbance experienced by individuals whose gender identity is incongruent with their biologic sex. "Transgender" refers to individuals whose gender identity is incongruent with their biological sex and others' perceptions of their gender, many of whom seek some degree of medical or surgical intervention to align their gender identity and anatomic phenotype. "Pansexual" is a recently used term to describe individuals who feel sexual attractions to all people, regardless of their gender. "LGBT" is a common acronym to describe lesbian, gay, bisexual, and transgender populations, although its use often categorizes individuals into 1 of 4 groupings, potentially excluding those who do not strictly identify along those lines. A broader term, "sexual minority youth," refers to any child or adolescent whose sexual orientation differs from that of the heterosexual norm, and may include those who identify as gay, bisexual, pansexual, or any other variation of a person's identified sexual attractions, arousal patterns, and sexual behaviors with another individual. "Gender-queer" is another recent term used by those who do not identify as fully male or fully female, but somewhere along the middle of the gender spectrum. "Gender minority youth" as opposed to "sexual minority youth" refers to any child or adolescent whose gender identity differs from that of the typical population where gender identity and biologic sex are usually concordant. This term broadly includes those youth who identify as transgender, gender nonconforming, and/or gender-queer. "Gender identity disorder" (GID) listed in the *Diagnostic and Statistical Manual of Mental Disorders*,[4] has 2 subtypes—childhood and adolescent/young adult—which currently requires individuals to meet a certain amount of criteria (depicting cross-gender expressions, behaviors, discomfort in an individual's anatomic sex) depending on the developmental timeframe during which the "symptoms" emerge. A subclinical diagnosis, Gender Identity Disorder Not Otherwise Specified (GID NOS), is reserved for individuals who may meet some criteria, yet do not meet the required amount necessary for the complete diagnosis. "Gender and sexuality competence" is an informal term created for use in this article to signify cultural competence pertaining to the provision of care for gender and sexual minorities specifically.

TREATMENT DISPARITY

Studies have historically highlighted the increased rates of psychopathology, including suicidal ideations and attempts, among lesbian, gay, and bisexual (LGB) youth compared to their straight counterparts.[5–7] More recently, factors related to increased risk for suicide in the transgender adolescent patient population were also explored.[8] Sexual minority youth who come from rejecting families are at an 8 times higher risk for suicide attempts compared to their counterparts from accepting families.[9] In addition to the marginalization and societal ostracism that gay, lesbian, and bisexual (sexual minority) youth typically experience, transgender adolescents also contend with gender dysphoria, an issue that often leads them to seek medical and surgical reassignment of their anatomic bodies. Others have described increased psychiatric comorbidity in children with GID as well.[10]

In 2009, the Massachusetts Youth Behavior Risk Survey reported that lesbian, gay, bisexual, and transgender (LGBT) youth are up to 4 times more likely to attempt suicide than are their heterosexual peers.[11] In 2009, the Gay and Lesbian Straight Education Network's (GLSEN) National School Climate Survey reported several alarming statistics[12]: (1) nearly 9 of 10 LGBT students experienced harassment in school; (2) increased levels of victimization were related to increased levels of depression and anxiety and decreased levels of self-esteem; (3) 61.1% of students reported that they felt unsafe in school because of their sexual orientation, and (4) 39.9% felt unsafe because of their gender expression. A recent study concluded that school victimization is a mediator for the development of poor psychosocial adjustment in gender nonconforming youth.[13] A recent review of suicide and suicidal risk in gender and sexual minority populations concluded that current mental health interventions, suicide prevention programs, and public policy did not sufficiently address the complexities of suicide research and prevention in these youth.[6]

With the lack of formal specialized interdisciplinary treatment programs, access to patient populations has been limited and research efforts to address these issues have been suboptimal. Articles have recently begun to highlight some of the dilemmas encountered: the lack of adequate classification of sexual minority youth, as many previously published surveys have not taken into account many youth who have had a same-sex experience but have not assumed a homosexual identity,[14] confounding previous results of youth surveys on suicide and other psychopathologies. Other barriers to research efforts to understand suicide risk factors in gender and sexual minority populations include difficulties studying "hidden populations"; historically sparse funding for these issues; and the omission of sexual orientation and gender identity from the broader sociodemographic characteristics that are routinely addressed in routine suicide and mental health studies.[6]

Despite the studies that highlight elevated risk for poor psychosocial adjustment in gender and sexual minority youths, only 1 study published in 1997 addresses how gay and lesbian issues are addressed in child and adolescent psychiatry training.[15] There have been no follow-up studies to address this issue since then, and other articles have highlighted numerous barriers to optimal health care between physicians and LGBT patients, regardless of physician specialty.[16,17] Additionally, there have been no published studies that describe how gender identity issues are addressed in child and adolescent psychiatry training programs. Recently, a study that evaluated the amount of hours devoted to LGBT issues in undergraduate medical education concluded that the major impediments to improved education as reported by faculty members were lack of instructional time, lack of relevance to their specific course content, and lack of professional development in that area.[18] Course directors who perceived these barriers were less likely to include these issues in the content of their teaching; however, it was also noted that advancement in faculty development could diminish those barriers.

Efforts to provide additional specialized interdisciplinary treatment programs for gender and sexual minority youth should be considered important and far-reaching.

GENDER MANAGEMENT SERVICE (GeMS) AT CHILDREN'S HOSPITAL BOSTON

The Division of Endocrinology at Children's Hospital Boston has provided medical management for the treatment of transgender adolescents (meeting criteria for GID; adolescent subtype) since 1998. In 2007, the Gender Management Service (GeMS) became a formalized treatment program operated jointly by the Divisions of Endocrinology and Urology to provide medical management for children with Disorders of Sex Development (DSD, otherwise known as intersex disorders. Shortly thereafter, interdisciplinary treatment was provided to adolescents with the diagnosis of GID and was accompanied by a 4-fold increase in the number of new patients per year. The inauguration of this service by the coauthor (N.P.S.) and pediatric urologist David Diamond, MD, represented the first such program in a U.S. children's hospital.

The GeMS program follows the published guidelines on the medical treatment of gender dysphoria in adolescents (S. Adelson and R.R. Pleak, personal communication, 2011).[2] Treatment involves both psychological and medical management over several different phases and is modeled after the "Dutch Protocol" (due to the fact that most of the research and clinical recommendations originated from the clinical and research experience of experts at the VU Medical Center in Amsterdam, the Netherlands). **Table 1** highlights the main aims in the psychosocial treatment aims in therapy according to the different phases of medical intervention. Ongoing psychosocial treatments in conjunction with a specialized battery of psychometric measures remain crucial components of the assessment for eligibility and readiness for medical interventions.[19,20]

The complex set of psychometric tests administered by the GeMS psychologist to assess readiness and eligibility have been consistently used in specialized gender treatment clinics in North America and Holland.[21,22] Testing formally assesses the degree of gender dysphoria, existence of comorbid psychiatric conditions, and psychosocial stability. For patients in the Tanner 2 or 3 puberty stages, timing of the assessment is essential given the irreversible progression of secondary sexual characteristics, which can be suppressed through hormonal interventions. The gender-specific measures used include the Recalled Childhood Gender Identity/Gender Role Questionnaire (RCGI),[23] the Body Image Scale,[24] the Gender Identity Interview for Adolescents (also known as the Gender Identity/Gender Dysphoria Questionnaire for Adolescents and Adults or the GIDYQ),[25] and the Utrecht Gender Dysphoria Scale.[26] Detailed descriptions of these measures is beyond the scope of

Table 1
Main goals of psychotherapy in gender nonconforming youth according to phase of treatment and developmental age

Stage of Treatment	Main Psychotherapeutic Aims
Prepubertal gender nonconforming children	Improve adaptive ego strengths and resilience in the child
	Facilitate parental understanding and support of the child
	Addess environmental factors that contribute to child invalidation
	Routine assessment of the degree of gender dysphoria persistence
	Address the current understanding of factors related to prepubertal cross-gender transition when appropriate
Pubertal gender nonconforming adolescent prehormonal intervention	Assess and clarify the diagnostic presentation by addressing the severity and/or intensification of gender dysphoria in the adolescent
	Assess readiness and eligibility criteria
	Facilitate a real-life experience while taking safety factors into account
	Educate regarding the effects of hormonal interventions
	Treat comorbid psychopathology within the context of gender identity
	Facilitate parental understanding and support of the adolescent and process
	Facilitate positive coping strategies to varying degrees of environmental invalidation
	Minimize components of environmental invalidation
Transgender adolescent receiving hormonal intervention	Facilitate adjustment to the physical changes of hormonal interventions
	Educate regarding the cross-gender transition and questions about surgical process
	Treat comorbid psychopathologies within the context of gender identity
	Facilitate parental understanding and support of the adolescent and process
	Facilitate appropriate positive coping strategies to varying degrees of environmental invalidation
	Address environmental factors that contribute to adolescent invalidation

Based on WPATH. The Harry Benjamin International Gender Dysphoria Association's Standards of Care for Gender Identity Disorders, Sixth Edition. Minneapolis, MN: 2001. Available at: http://www.wpath.org. Accessed July 14, 2011.

this article. These have been described in descriptive studies on the clinical management of gender identity disorder.[21] Other measures that are more commonly used to assess global psychopathologies include the Child Behavior Check List (CBCL),[27] the Children's Depression Inventory (CDI),[28] the Revised Children's Manifest Anxiety Scale (RCMAS),[29] Youth Self-Report form (YSR),[27] Conners ADHD scales,[30] and the Aspergers Syndrome Diagnostic Scale (ASDS).[31]

The psychometric testing typically takes 6 to 8 hours to complete and can only be provided to a maximum of 2 patients monthly. The GeMS child and adolescent psychologist is trained to incorporate the results of these testing measures with the narrative report from patient and family members and a letter of referral from the treating mental health clinician to assess eligibility for the commencement of hormonal interventions.

The medical interventions are largely determined by the pubertal stage. For adolescents at Tanner Stage 2 to 3, pubertal suppression through use of GnRH analogues is used to reversibly prevent the development of unwanted secondary sexual characteristics of the natal sex. This was first investigated in the Amsterdam Clinic for Children and Adolescents in 2000, and subsequent follow-up studies have confirmed that psychosocial adjustment improved through use of this intervention.[19,32–34] Ultimately, the use of partially irreversible cross-sex hormones (testosterone for natal females and estrogen for natal males) produces secondary sexual characteristics of the individual's affirmed gender once their social, cognitive, and emotional development mature and an informed decision can be made about the physical changes that will happen. For adolescents presenting in the later Tanner stages (4 and 5), pubertal suppression has less benefit and cross-sex hormones are the first-line medical intervention. There is a growing consensus that use of pubertal suppression in these individuals may actually require less cross-sex hormone dosing to achieve the same desired effect with decreased propensity for the development of unwanted side effects from the cross-sex hormones themselves.

The original GeMS program offered medical interventions exclusively to youth seeking gender transition, and the patient population it serviced had been limited to those who fulfilled the criteria for these types of interventions–adolescents who have already entered puberty and were at Tanner stage 2 or higher. At the time of inception in 2007, GeMS was staffed to provide both psychometric testing by the GeMS child and adolescent psychologist as well as the medical interventions by a pediatric endocrinologist. Notably lacking from the program was an in-house psychiatric service to provide ongoing mental health treatment for its patients and the prepubescent gender nonconforming children who were seeking providers. Consistent with the experience in other international gender clinics, patients were presenting with increasingly more complex comorbid psychiatric diagnoses,[10,35,36] and psychopharmacologic interventions were also unavailable. Without another specialized gender clinic for adolescents in New England, many patients have traveled vast geographic distances to obtain services not often provided in their local communities. **Box 1** describes the hurdles in more detail.

Box 1
Identified barriers to providing competent comprehensive care for gender nonconforming youth in the absence of an in-house psychiatric service when providing medical services to transgender adolescents

- Lack of services for prepubescent children not requiring hormonal interventions
- Lack of psychopharmacologic interventions for complex comorbid psychiatric presentations
- Difficulty establishing consistent ongoing contact with a multitude of community providers
- Variability of community provider comfort regarding gender identity issues
- Variability of community provider knowledge regarding the standards of care for gender nonconforming youth
- Lack of obtaining standardized psychiatric measures to determine the severity and classification of associated psychopathologies

Prior to the establishment of a formal psychiatric counterpart service to ensure that the ongoing psychiatric needs of patients were met, the GeMS team relied on the services of outside community providers who were variably experienced with the needs of the patient population (specified by the WPATH guidelines). Determining the varying levels of expertise of these outside clinicians remained logistically impossible for the team given the lack of any formal ability to assess any clinician's "gender competence." For the in-house providers, the requirement to establish ongoing contact with a multitude of outside clinicians often resulted in numerous, cumbersome attempts to gather information about the ongoing psychosocial aspects of care. Interactions were frequently made through written forms of communication, which lacked the necessary assessment of an outside provider's comfort and awareness of the complex treatment issues involved. When telephone conversations were possible, logistical barriers may have resulted in brief conversations that would sometimes focus more on the therapist's knowledge of gender identity issues versus the individual clinical needs of the patient. The lack of adequate consistency and coordination of care remained an impediment to optimal systematic interdisciplinary treatment.

DEVELOPMENT OF THE PSYCHOSOCIAL GENDER IDENTITY CLINIC
Demographics of the Patient Population and Clinical Modalities Provided

Since its formal creation in 2007, the GeMS program at Children's Hospital Boston was in a unique position to offer interdisciplinary services for transgender adolescents by providing mental health treatment in conjunction with hormone therapies. In October 2009, GeMS referred its first patient for ongoing psychosocial treatment to an in-house child and adolescent psychiatry resident (coauthor S.L.) in the Department of Psychiatry. Since then, an ongoing collaboration has developed, serving the needs of 23 patients (as of May 2011), one day per week by the same clinician, now a junior faculty psychiatrist (S.L.). This collaboration marked the first time that an academic children's hospital in the United States offered systematic interdisciplinary services for all gender minority youth. The presenting patients have represented a wide spectrum of developmental stages, comorbid psychopathologies, sociodemographic characteristics, and treatment needs. **Figs. 1** and **2** display the developmental stages, natal sex, and GID diagnostic classifications of the patients at the time of their initial presentation over the first 18 months of service. Many logistical considerations have impacted the provision of care for these minority youth. **Table 2** displays the type of treatment service initially sought by patients as differentiated by their developmental stage. Future sections of this article will explore these treatment services and other issues relevant to the development of a specialized gender (and sexuality) psychosocial clinic while taking into account the treatment and logistical considerations.

To date, the patient age at the time of presentation for psychiatric evaluation and treatment has ranged from 5 to 22 years. An overwhelming majority of referrals have been provided through the GeMS intake process, coordinated by the GeMS social worker. All but 2 of the referred patients resided within a 60-mile radius of the Boston metropolitan area. Additionally, all but 1 presented with chief complaints of "gender-nonconforming behaviors and/or identifications." While a substantial majority of the patients have been referred through the GeMS program intake process, only 5 patients receiving psychiatric treatment in the specialized clinic actually received medical hormone interventions through GeMS at the time of writing. Several patients have received ongoing psychiatric treatment to address the impairments in mental

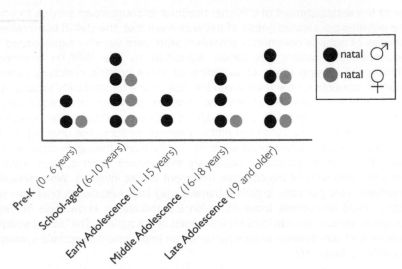

Fig. 1. Number of patients in each stage of development, differentiated by natal sex at initial presentation.

health functioning that would preclude them from being eligible for hormonal interventions.

An overview of the services provided for these patients in the specialized gender clinic is displayed in **Box 2**. Patients presenting for treatment were categorized into those seeking one time consultation versus those seeking ongoing treatment services

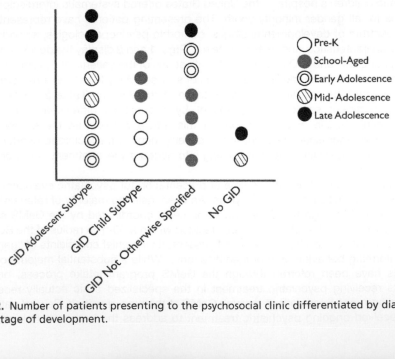

Fig. 2. Number of patients presenting to the psychosocial clinic differentiated by diagnosis and stage of development.

Table 2
Number of patients presenting for psychiatric treatment differentiated by stage of development and type of initially sought treatment service

	Patients Seeking One-Time Consultation	Patients Seeking Ongoing Treatment	Patients Seeking Exclusive Treatment in the Specialized Treatment Program	Patients Seeking Psychosocial Treatment in Collaboration with an Outside Clinician
Pre-K (0–6 years)	0	3	2	1
School-aged (6–10 years)	1	6	5	1
Early adolescence (11–15 years)	1	4	1	3
Middle adolescence (16–18 years)	1	3	2	1
Late adolescence (19 and older)	2	2	1	1

Box 2
Types of current services provided in the Gender Identity Psychosocial Clinic

- Comprehensive psychiatric services within the specialty clinic (psychosocial and psychopharmacologic treatment)
- Psychopharmacology services in collaboration with an outside psychosocial therapy partner
- Periodic gender identity consultation with an outside psychosocial therapy provider
- One-time gender identity consultation with an outside psychiatric provider

---

in some capacity. For patients seeking continued treatment services, one of three types of services have been provided: full treatment in the gender specialty clinic (psychotherapy and psychopharmacologic treatment, when appropriate), psychopharmacology services in collaboration with an outside psychosocial therapy provider, and periodic psychosocial "gender-specific" consultation in collaboration with an outside provider. Eighteen of the 23 patients have received ongoing services in the treatment clinic, while five presented for a one time consultation. Of those 18 patients, 11 received full treatment within the specialty clinic, while seven have been in collaboration with an outside provider. Three of those patients in collaboration have received psychopharmacologic interventions through the specialized clinic, while the 4 other patients have only required periodic consultation in collaboration with a previously established outside provider regarding the gender identity issues. Detailed analysis of the contributing demographic factors associated with treatment-modality decisions is beyond the scope of this article given the lack of a sufficient population sample necessary to infer significant conclusions.

The families of the gender nonconforming children (2 natal males and 1 natal female) who presented prior to the start of kindergarten had questions about the benefits of assuming a cross-gender social role in the school setting. Seven school-aged children of ages ranging from 6 to 9 (including 3 gender nonconforming females) were referred for consultation or ongoing treatment. Five early pubertal adolescents presented for treatment (all natal males), with 4 continuing to receive services in the specialized clinic. Three of those 4 have been in collaboration with an outside provider.

Eight of the patients initially assessed were natal females, while 15 were natal males, yet only 60% of the prepubertal children were natal males. This differs from the existing literature that suggests an overwhelming majority of prepubertal children presenting with gender nonconforming behaviors and identifications are typically natal males.[37] The small sample size of the patient population limits the ability to draw significant conclusions on this issue.

For the prepubertal children, in addition to carrying diagnoses of GID (either the childhood subtype or NOS), other diagnosed Axis I disorders at the time of assessment included pervasive developmental disorder, attention-deficit/hyperactivity disorder; combined type, adjustment disorder with mixed disturbance of conduct and emotions, generalized anxiety disorder, depressive disorder NOS, and adjustment disorder with mixed anxiety and depression. For the early-, middle-, and late-stage adolescents, initial assessments revealed major depressive disorder, cannabis abuse, panic disorder, Asperger's disorder, and obsessive-compulsive disorder as comorbid diagnoses. Several patients referred for assessment did not meet the full criteria for GID, childhood or adolescent/young adult subtype, but rather GID NOS (see **Fig. 2**), and 2 patients did not meet criteria for any form of GID.

Prioritization of Psychometric Testing

The addition of a specialized psychiatric treatment service in the Department of Psychiatry alleviates several logistical challenges previously experienced by the GeMS team when mental health services solely consisted of bimonthly psychometric testing. More readily available, initial psychiatric evaluations are completed in 2 hours and can be offered on a weekly basis. For patients with complex psychiatric comorbidities, psychiatric consultation may determine that scheduling the psychometric testing should be delayed, helping prioritize the time-sensitive testing for other patients who may meet readiness and eligibility criteria sooner. Direct weekly communication between the social worker, psychiatrist, and psychologist helps ensure that patients' mental health needs are met both in terms of timing and complexity.

Milieu and Documentation Considerations

Several other logistical issues have come to the forefront with respect to providing care in an academic medical center to gender minority youth. Published guidelines have addressed some of these milieu considerations for gender nonconforming individuals in medical settings.[38]

Shortly after the routine presence of gender minority youth in the outpatient psychiatry clinic, it became apparent that office staff needed to be aware of patients' chosen names, which often did not correspond to the name listed in the medical record depending on whether the patient's name had been legally changed. This required constant interaction between clinicians and office staff to minimize awkward patient encounters at the front desk or in the waiting room.

All staff members have developed a heightened sense of awareness regarding the climate of the patient waiting room, which typically serves a variety of patients and families representing diverse ethnic, social, and developmental demographics. Many of these patients and families have been observed inadvertently (or blatantly) staring at patients whose phenotypic gender expression is ambiguous. Depending on the adaptive ego-strengths of the gender nonconforming or transgender patient, subtle interactions have been perceived as invalidating or uncomfortable.

For patients requiring psychotropic medication prescriptions whose names have not been formally changed in the medical record, a printout of the prescription from the electronic medical record (with the legal natal name listed) can lead to discomfort or anguish. Understanding the impact that this may have on a patient's adherence to a medication regimen has yet to be explored, yet an open discussion that addresses the patient's feelings about having their natal name (and sex) on the prescription bottle has been effective at putting the patient and family at ease. Although some patients and families may never see the medical record, documentation remains another issue for institutions whose records exclusively allow for 1 of 2 gender options: male or female. Documentation that prevents a clinician from distinguishing natal sex from affirmed gender identity may force a clinician to choose a category that does not accurately describe the clinical status of the patient. Additionally, this binary choice excludes those patients who affirm a gender identity that is neither exclusively male nor female.

Several patients and families have reported that clinician acknowledgment of these issues displays an empathic understanding of the patient's ongoing distress, which ultimately enhanced flexibility and adaptation to these perceived environmental injustices.

Measuring Clinical Effectiveness

Developing a specialized treatment service in an academic hospital setting demands a capacity to measure clinical effectiveness. The use of rating scales and psychometric instruments is necessary for both the provision of competent clinical care and development of research initiatives. Determining the usefulness of each of these scales at various points in the treatment has required ongoing collaboration with the GeMS psychologist. The choice and frequency of scale administration depends on numerous factors including developmental stage of the patient, type of presenting problem, and detailed knowledge of the specific measures of gender dysphoria obtained routinely by psychologists in the field. Measures administered should assess broader categories of psychopathology (CBCL, YSR,[27] depressive scales such as the CDI[28] or CES-D,[39] anxiety scales such as the RCMAS,[31] and an ADHD assessment such as the Conners scale[30]) in addition to gender-specific domains (gender dysphoria and gender identity development) including the Draw-a-Person test,[40–42] Body Image Scale,[24] Recalled Childhood Gender Identity/Gender Role Questionnaire (RCGI),[23] and Utrecht Gender Dysphoria Scale[26] used by the GeMS psychologist when determining eligibility and readiness for medical interventions.

CLINICAL AND ETHICAL ISSUES IN THE PSYCHOSOCIAL TREATMENT OF GENDER MINORITY YOUTH

For prepubertal gender nonconforming children, understanding the psychosexual outcomes of development raises ethical and treatment issues. The current scientific understanding of gender nonconforming behaviors in children lacks any definitive means to accurately predict the persistence or desistance of gender nonconforming identifications and behaviors into adolescence.[43] The prospective studies on gender nonconforming children all show that the overwhelming majority of these children will ultimately desist from their cross-gender identifications and behaviors by adolescence.[32,33,44–46] The data also suggest that a majority of these children will identify as sexual minorities as they become adolescents. More recent research has attempted to determine whether the "severity" of gender dysphoria in children is more predictive of the persistence of these feelings into adolescence,[33] yet the current diagnostic classification of GID remains vague in its ability to define "severity." Distinguishing between the gender nonconforming children who persist with an insistence that they are the opposite gender from those who do not remains the area of focus for experts reclassifying the diagnosis in the DSM-5.[47–49]

The lack of evidence-based treatment options for the approach to a gender nonconforming child confounds the ethical and clinical dilemmas outlined by experts. Three general approaches can be taken[43]: reducing the gender dysphoria through cognitive and behavioral strategies (eg, attempting to increase the child's comfort by expressing behaviors and identifications consistent with his/her natal sex); redirecting the child to neutral expressions of gender in an attempt by allowing more time for the child to develop cognitively, emotionally, and socially; or facilitating an ego-syntonic cross-gender social transition prior to the onset of puberty. Each of these approaches has its associated benefits and risks, and therefore reclassifying the GID diagnosis in the DSM-5 may enhance future evidence-based studies to determine which approach best meets the needs for a given child.

Parents with younger gender nonconforming children often seek definitive answers about the future outcome of their child when he or she identifies as the opposite sex. Parents often feel forced to balance the conflict between validating their child's current stated wishes versus succumbing to the stigma that their environmental influences (family members, friends, educators, acquaintances, etc) may impose. They may question whether their current decisions might influence a particular outcome in the future. To balance those needs, the parents may seek to rely on the expertise of a professional to assist them in determining the best approach to managing competing demands.

For the clinician, parallel ethical conflicts may arise.[50] Determining the extent to which specific directives in day-to-day management may reinforce parental reliance on the clinician. It may not be in the best interest of the child or family to increase reliance on the clinician for answers. Also, given the high desistance rates of gender-nonconforming behaviors and identifications in children, facilitating a prepubertal cross-gender social transition is a highly complex issue without much evidence to inform standardized practice.[43,51] Addressing concerns that the treatment recommendations may actually influence the outcome of the child's gender identity is an ongoing conflict for many clinicians who specifically choose to work with these children. A clinician with specific expertise in gender identity must assess the recommendations of other providers (pediatrician, school psychologist, teacher, therapist, etc) involved in the treatment of a child—some of which may develop from inadvertent (or blatant) opposing ideas and biases.

The evidence-based treatment options for gender nonconforming (some meeting criteria for GID NOS) and transgender adolescents (GID, adolescent subtype) are more available than for gender nonconforming children. However, given the lack of comfort that many, if not most, mental health clinicians report when dealing with gender identity issues, determining a specific patient's eligibility and readiness for treatment may be inconsistent across providers. Psychosocial treatment for adolescents who present as gender nonconforming is necessary for a variety of reasons. These include the ability to provide diagnostic assessment, determine a particular adolescent's adaptive ego strengths, facilitate the initiation of medical interventions when necessary, and improve adaptation to the many possible external and internal challenges experienced by the adolescent.

The various medical interventions outlined in this article require an in-depth understanding by mental health practitioners when providing concurrent psychosocial treatment. The clinician must understand that the distress experienced by a transgender adolescent whose body begins to develop secondary sexual characteristics (of their natal sex) is necessary for the diagnosis of GID, adolescent subtype. While GnRH analogues reversibly delay the onset of these characteristics, not all families may be willing to undergo the logistical hurdles that present when seeking expensive treatments not routinely covered by insurance. This may contribute to an adolescent's perception that his or her parents are unsupportive or rejecting. This may also prevent supportive parents of lesser means from being able to appropriately tend to their adolescent's treatment needs.

The initiation of cross-sex hormone therapy at around the age of 16 presents other considerations and barriers to optimal treatment. While less expensive, these interventions create physical changes that are partially irreversible. Understanding the effects on the human reproductive system should be explored in therapy prior to their initiation, which provides education to the adolescent (and family) about sperm or egg preservation for future reproduction. A clinician should be aware of the expected and unexpected changes that come with exogenous cross-sex hormone administration. The clinician must facilitate patient adjustment to the varying degrees of environmental invalidation as his or her physical characteristics change. Knowing the legal rights and protective laws in a particular state or country is essential when providing effective treatment to an adolescent undergoing the physical changes of gender transition. Finally, a clinician must involve the adolescent's parents into the treatment decisions given the age of legal consent.

CLINICAL TREATMENT MODALITY OPTIONS

Establishing a treatment plan that optimally meets the needs of the child and family can present barriers and challenges. Considering the lack of specialized treatment programs for gender identity and sexuality, patients and families often come from distant geographic locations, which may limit the possibility of establishing an ongoing psychosocial treatment relationship that incorporates regular follow-up treatment sessions. At the time of presentation, parents may be seeking consultation (1-time assessments) for treatment issues that often require ongoing follow-up visits. Therefore, an initial assessment can be categorized into one of two types of services: a one-time consultation versus the establishment of an ongoing treatment frame (**Box 2**).

One-Time Consultation Versus Ongoing Treatment Frame

The benefits and limitations of the type of psychiatric service sought by families in a specialized gender identity clinic are portrayed in **Tables 3** and **4**, respectively. The purpose of the consultation may be helpful to families who already have an established mental health treatment provider, yet feel that further clarification of the differential diagnosis and treatment outcomes of gender nonconforming behavior is needed. With the establishment of an ongoing treatment relationship, it may be possible for the clinician to assume complete responsibility for the mental health treatment or join a collaborative frame with a variety of providers, each providing a specific role.

Given the time-dependent nature of gender and sexual development in the context of a child's broader cognitive, emotional, social, and behavioral development, clarification that a one time consultation has limitations is crucial. However, the clinician providing a one time consultation for a child may be able to facilitate understanding of the following: (1) assessment of parental intentions with respect to their child's day-to-day behaviors; (2) assessment of parental expectations of their child's future gender development trajectory; (3) diagnostic clarification of the child's presentation (GID: childhood subtype versus subclinical GID NOS); (4) assessment of the extent to which the current treatment plan in place (if one exists) addresses the gender identity issues; (5) assessment of any co-morbid psychiatric diagnoses; (6) initial assessment of the environmental influences on the child's gender development (school, peers, extended family members, siblings, popular culture, etc); (7) provision of psychoeducation and resources; and (8) intervention when safety is compromised. With an adolescent, an additional benefit of a one time consultation includes the ability to assess priority for psychometric testing, the step required for medical hormone intervention.

A one time consultation for a child may not be able to offer recommendations for the following issues: (1) specific guidance regarding the child's future trajectory; (2) detailed understanding of the complex interactions between gender development and other co-morbid psychiatric conditions; (3) patterns of the child's coping strategies and resilience capacities; (4) detailed understanding of the interplaying environmental factors and their relationships to the child's gender and sexual development; and (5) limited ability to provide long-term intervention when a child's environment is particularly invalidating. For an adolescent, an additional limitation is the ability to provide psychiatric clearance for medical hormone interventions if necessary.

The establishment of an ongoing treatment relationship expands the possibilities to understand the dynamic interaction between psychiatric co-morbidities, various

Table 3
Benefits of the type of psychiatric treatment service provided in a specialized interdisciplinary gender identity psychosocial clinic differentiated by stage of development

	One-Time Consultation	Ongoing Treatment
Prepubescent Children	• May clarify initial parental intentions for child's treatment	• All the benefits of a one-time consultation
	• May clarify parental expectations of child's future trajectory	• More complex understanding of the interactions between comorbidities, external influences, internal ego strengths, and gender identity issues
	• Diagnostic clarification of gender identity issues	• Ability to provide treatment for comorbid psychiatric diagnoses
	• Ability to assess the extent that the current treatment measures address the gender identity issues	• Ability to provide ongoing support for the child through the therapeutic treatment relationship
	• Ability to assess comorbid psychiatric diagnoses	• Ability to provide ongoing support for a child's family through the therapeutic treatment relationship
	• Ability to obtain initial assessment of environmental factors on adolescent's gender development	
	• Provision of psychoeducation and resources	
	• May be useful for an outside provider seeking consultation	
	• May provide short-term intervention when safety is compromised	
Adolescents	• May clarify initial parental intentions for adolescent's treatment	• All the benefits of a one-time consultation
	• May clarify parental expectations of adolescent's future trajectory	• More complex understanding of the interactions between comorbidities, external influences, internal ego strengths, and gender identity issues
	• Diagnostic clarification of gender identity issues	• Ability to provide treatment for comorbid psychiatric diagnoses
	• Ability to assess the extent that the current treatment measures address the gender identity issues	• Ability to provide ongoing support for an adolescent through the therapeutic treatment relationship
	• Ability to assess comorbid psychiatric diagnoses	• Ability to provide ongoing support for an adolescent's family through the therapeutic treatment relationship
	• Ability to obtain initial assessment of environmental factors on adolescent's gender development	
	• Provision of psychoeducation and resources	
	• May be useful for an outside provider seeking consultation	
	• May provide short-term intervention when safety is compromised	

Table 4
Limitations of the type of psychiatric treatment service provided in a specialized interdisciplinary gender identity psychosocial clinic differentiated by stage of development

	One-Time Consultation	Ongoing Treatment
Prepubescent Children	• Inability to predict the future trajectory of child's gender and sexual development • Limited ability to understand the complex interaction between gender development and other associated comorbid psychiatric conditions • Limited ability to understand ongoing patterns of resilience and coping strategies for the particular child • Limited ability to understand the time-dependent interplay between environmental factors and the child's gender and sexual development • Limited ability to provide long-term intervention when determining a child's environment is particularly invalidating	• Variability in the amount of time it takes to clarify the trajectory of the child's gender and/or sexual development • Lack of standardized measures that can be used to quantify the relative degree of stress that each environmental factor has on the child's gender development • Logistical difficulties that may limit the frequency of treatment sessions (travel, insurance)
Adolescents	• Inability to provide clearance for medical treatment interventions if needed • Limited ability to understand the complex interaction between gender development and other associated comorbid psychiatric conditions • Limited ability to understand ongoing patterns of resilience and coping strategies for the particular adolescent • Limited ability to understand the time-dependent interplay between environmental factors and the adolescent's gender and sexual development • Limited ability to provide long-term intervention when determining an adolescent's environment is particularly invalidating	• Variability in the amount of time it takes to determine eligibility and readiness criteria for a particular adolescent • Lack of standardized measures that can be used to quantify the relative degree of stress that each environmental factor has on the adolescent's gender development • Difficulties arising from adolescent's potential age-appropriate resistance to therapy • Logistical difficulties that may limit the frequency of treatment sessions (travel, insurance)

external influences on the child or adolescent, internal ego strengths and coping patterns, and the gender identity questions at hand. The timeframe with which these details emerge may be different based on the individual characteristics of the patient and family. Despite the advantage of establishing a long-term treatment relationship several limitations exist in this treatment frame. Depending on the presenting age of a child, it may take several years before conclusions can be drawn regarding the persistence or desistence of the gender nonconforming behaviors and identifications. Quantifying the relative degree that each environmental influence may have on the development of the individual gender nonconforming child's comorbid psychopathologies remains a challenge given the lack of standardized measures to assess varying degrees of environmental invalidation. For adolescents, an age-appropriate resistance to therapy sometimes presents in the treatment frame often due to the adolescent's perception that they are well-adjusted and do not require psychosocial follow-up while taking cross-sex hormones. For both children and adolescents, logistical considerations (travel distance, insurance issues, etc) may present as barriers when establishing an ongoing treatment service in a specialized clinic.

The decision to assume complete responsibility for the child or adolescent's mental health treatment largely rests upon two factors: feasibility for parents to adhere to the recommended frequency of visits and the possibility of obtaining competent care from a community provider who may or may not have knowledge of the complex treatment issues at hand. The frequency of treatment is guided by the severity of associated psychopathology and degree of functioning. In some situations, these pathologies are quickly alleviated with intensive short-term therapy focusing on self-esteem, resilience, and enhancing adaptive ego strengths,[52] yet a longer course of increased frequency of visits may be needed for others. For families electing to receive their child's complete psychiatric care at the specialized center, a discussion about the feasibility of adherence to a recommended frequency of visits would be important during the initial psychiatric assessment.

Collaborative Treatment with a Community Provider

For families willing to enter an ongoing treatment frame with two different mental health providers in place, several steps should be taken to determine if the child or adolescent's ongoing mental health needs would be met. A collaborative discussion with the community provider should include a discussion about the treatment aims, determination of the outside provider's individual comfort level regarding gender nonconforming behaviors and identifications, and proposed frequency of follow-up visits. Visits in a specialized treatment clinic may be less frequent, yet still enhance the overall mental health treatment by providing ongoing recommendations and support to community providers. External barriers to care (such as insurance coverage) should be explored to determine the possibility of having two mental health providers in place, and subsequent ability for parents to carry financial responsibility in the event that insurance logistics render that possibility unfeasible. Finally, periodic discussions between providers should be maintained to address the clinical issues of the patient as they unfold.

INTERDISCIPLINARY COOPERATION AND THE GeMS REFERRAL PROCESS

Medical-psychiatric collaboration for the treatment of transgender adolescents is a necessity yet few endocrinology or child and adolescent psychiatry training programs have access to the patient population in a specialized interdisciplinary clinic. The establishment of both medical and psychiatric services that specifically tend to gender identity and transition within a single academic institution remains critical for the future treatment of gender minority youth across the developmental spectrum. Understanding the day-to-day logistical issues may alleviate the burden of ignorance that often prevents the development and creation of new "gender identity specific" services.

When a family seeks GeMS services, the program coordinator refers the parent to the GeMS social worker who performs an initial phone intake to obtain an overview of the patient's specific needs, both psychiatric and medical. The protocol is explained to families seeking information about treatment options. For those seeking hormonal treatments, the social worker explains the need for patients to have ongoing counseling with a mental health provider who could ultimately be expected to write a referral letter that substantiates the patient's persistence of cross-gender affirmation and identity. Patients not receiving mental health care may be referred for an initial psychiatric assessment in the psychosocial gender identity clinic within the Department of Psychiatry, depending on the previously discussed logistical considerations (location and insurance). Patients with established mental health treatment are referred for additional psychiatric assessment to address the specific gender identity issues when an outside clinician seeks clarification.

Weekly rounds are attended by the GeMS team: the pediatric endocrinologist, child and adolescent psychiatrist, child and adolescent psychologist, staff social worker, and program coordinator. Several clinical matters are routinely addressed: review of new patient inquiries with proper disposition planning, discussion of patients scheduled for psychometric testing, review of patients scheduled for medical follow-up visits, and complex issues arising for existing patients that require interdisciplinary discussion, and other logistical concerns (including insurance barriers and scheduling priorities).

Patients and families often view the mental health component of treatment as a means to achieving their medical interventions. In many instances, patients display poor adherence to mental health follow-up visits once achieving their primary goal: hormonal interventions and/or a referral letter for sexual reassignment surgery. In an attempt to maximize patient adherence to the psychosocial component of treatment, the GeMS team developed a standardized form to be filled out by parents at all medical visits. It requests information regarding the last appointment scheduled with a mental health professional, recent changes in psychiatric medications or mental health providers, and any recent changes in the child or adolescent's psychiatric functioning. The form is filled out at their medical visit, and is reviewed by the medical provider (endocrinologist) to address any changes in treatment that may have occurred since the previous appointment. The GeMS social worker subsequently reviews the information and performs a more detailed follow-up assessment when necessary. In the event that acute safety issues (possibly requiring acute psychiatric hospitalization) are revealed, patients are immediately referred to the emergency room for a more thorough psychiatric assessment. For those patients requiring less acute interventions, the GeMS social worker provides additional psycho-education to families regarding the importance of ongoing mental health visits. Further assessment may determine other barriers to optimal mental health treatment including insurance issues, poor "therapist-patient fit," suboptimal focus on gender issues within therapy, suboptimal clinician comfort when discussing gender identity issues, and/or any additional logistical barriers to receiving ongoing care (location, transportation, scheduling, etc).

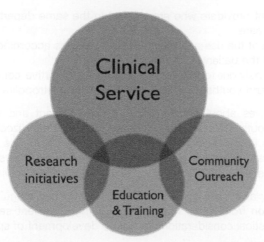

Fig. 3. Relationship between clinical, research, education, and community domains when promoting institutional gender competence. In an academic medical center, the opportunities to expand research development, community outreach, and broader training/education initiatives are contingent on the development of clinical services, which provides a patient population base.

FUTURE INITIATIVES

Efforts to improve the treatment of gender and sexual minority youth requires expansion of clinical services, research initiatives, training and education, and community outreach. To address the gender and sexuality competence gap among health providers in North America, institutions must foment more partnerships between medical and psychiatric departments to provide specialized comprehensive care for these youth.

Broadening these services requires physicians and mental health clinicians to become familiar with the treatment issues and logistical considerations involved in developing interdisciplinary collaborative services. Doing so is both feasible and necessary, given the proven disparities in access to optimal health care experienced by gender and sexual minority youth. In an academic medical center, the opportunities to expand research development, community outreach, and broader training/education initiatives are contingent upon the development of clinical services, which provides a patient population base. **Fig. 3** depicts the reliance that expansion of these three domains has on clinical care. An endocrinologist or adolescent medicine specialist eager to evaluate and treat these patients is a prerequisite.

With the growth of the patient population seeking treatment in the specialized treatment clinic—evidenced by the substantial growth of the patient population in the GeMS program in its first years of operation—demand for clinical services may require expansion in the following areas:

1. Group therapy services that serve the needs of its patients and families while taking into account the appropriate clinical issues across all developmental stages.
2. Family therapy services to address the varying issues that arise in families of gender nonconforming youths.
3. Parental support treatments that can be provided concurrently with the individual treatments offered for their youth, which facilitates improved communication

among treatment providers who are located in the same department, enhancing competency of care.

4. Standardization of the use and timing of rating scales according to the developmental stage of the patient.
5. Online support network to facilitate appropriate supportive communications between families and youths residing within a specific metropolitan region.

Research initiatives about gender atypical development and the treatment of gender minority youth are currently relegated to few specialized interdisciplinary treatment centers in the world (Toronto and Amsterdam). The development of statistically significant prospective study designs relies upon large sample sizes. The contributions to research efforts that may result include the following:

1. Efforts to study and classify initial parental intentions distinguishing those who seek consultation from those requesting ongoing treatment services. This may also inform logistical considerations for future development of specialized gender identity clinics.
2. Efforts to study and classify treatment outcomes when distinguishing between parents initially seeking consultation from those requesting ongoing treatment services. This may also inform logistical considerations for the future development of specialized gender identity clinics.
3. Studies of the potential mediators of psychotropic medication compliance in gender minority youth populations.
4. Further contribution to efforts that study the predictability of the persistence of gender dysphoria and nonconforming behaviors from childhood into adolescence.
5. Development of measures that accurately assess the severity of gender dysphoria (ie, severity of anatomic rejection of natal genitalia) in gender nonconforming prepubertal children.
6. Development of measures that can standardize and quantify the degrees of environmental invalidation experienced by gender and sexual minority youths.

The gap in education and training, both within the sphere of psychiatry and the health care industry at large, remains an ongoing impediment to providing universal gender-competent care for gender (and sexual) minority youths. Detailed assessment of these issues are explored elsewhere in this volume,[53] but the development of an interdisciplinary specialized gender identity clinic in an academic institution creates opportunities that can ultimately enhance the implementation of the following measures:

1. Improving faculty development across specialties designed to enhance the supervision of residents and other trainees about gender identity and sexuality.
2. Facilitating patient referrals to residents and other trainees to broaden their experience when dealing with these issues early on in their careers.
3. Including gender identity and sexuality in case conferences, didactic instruction, and grand round presentations.
4. Training psychologists on the sophisticated psychometrics of gender identity measurements.
5. Fomenting interdisciplinary cooperation between medical, psychiatry, psychology, and social work training programs.

While the development of a specialized treatment clinic promotes expansion of clinical services, research developments, and education initiatives, addressing these issues within the context of an academic institution lacks immediate benefit for community providers unaffiliated with a formal medical school or training program. Outreach to local agencies and community providers should be considered in the development objectives for any specialized treatment clinic that serves gender and sexual minority youth. These goals can ultimately address the following issues:

1. Providing seminars and supervisory roles to clinicians in the community who are seeking support from academic institutions with respect to developing "gender and sexuality competence."
2. Unifying health care providers against discriminatory legislation that currently exist in many states and countries against gender and sexual minorities.
3. Improving the provision of care to underserved populations who often seek treatment in community centers accepting alternative insurance policies.
4. Enhancing research initiatives through increased access to patient populations and larger sample sizes when designing prospective studies.

SUMMARY

The existing treatment gap for gender and sexual minority youths will widen if concrete steps to emphasize the importance of "gender and sexuality competence" are not taken. Academic institutions with formal training programs are in a unique position at the crossroads of clinical, research, education, and community initiatives to serve the needs of these youth. Access to clinical care is a prerequisite for the development of the other components, and it is crucial that academic institutions prioritize the creation of specific services that serve marginalized populations, who often feel they have no place to turn. Doing so is feasible, yet requires understanding of the clinical, logistical, and interdisciplinary issues.

Competent providers not only benefit the patients who seek them, but the institutions with whom they are affiliated, the researchers who need large clinical samples with standardized treatment approaches, and the broader community who may unknowingly perpetuate the prevailing culture of discrimination against gender and sexual minority youth that still exists today.

ACKNOWLEDGMENTS

The authors acknowledge Enrico Mezzacappa, MD, Laura Edwards-Leeper, PhD, Francie Mandel, LICSW, Sarah Dobbins, and Kimberly Withrow.

REFERENCES

1. National Residency Match Program. Results and data: specialties matching service 2010 appointment year. Washington, DC: National Residency Match Program; 2010. Available at: http://www.nrmp.org. Accessed July 14, 2011.
2. Hembree WC, Cohen-Kettenis P, Delemarre-van de Waal HA, et al. Endocrine treatment of transsexual persons: an Endocrine Society clinical practice guideline. J Clin Endocrinol Metab 2009;94(9):3132–54.
3. WPATH. The Harry Benjamin International Gender Dysphoria Association's standards of care for gender identity disorders. 6th edition. Minneapolis (MN): 2001:22. Available at: http://www.wpath.org. Accessed July 14, 2011.
4. American Psychiatric Association. Diagnostic and statistical manual of mental disorders. 4th edition. Washington, DC: American Psychiatric Association Press; 1994.
5. Savin-Williams RC, Ream GL. Suicide attempts among sexual-minority male youth. J Clin Child Adolesc Psychol 2003;32(4):509–22.

6. Haas AP, Eliason M, Mays VM, et al. Suicide and suicide risk in lesbian, gay, bisexual, and transgender populations: review and recommendations. J Homosex 2011;58(1): 10–51.

7. Remafedi G, French S, Story M, et al. The relationship between suicide risk and sexual orientation: results of a population-based study. Am J Public Health 1998;88(1):57–60.

8. Grossman AH, D'Augelli AR. Transgender youth and life-threatening behaviors. Suicide Life Threat Behav 2007;37(5):527–37.

9. Ryan C, Huebner D, Diaz RM, et al. Family rejection as a predictor of negative health outcomes in white and Latino lesbian, gay, and bisexual young adults. Pediatrics 2009;123(1):346–52.

10. Wallien MS, Swaab H, Cohen-Kettenis PT. Psychiatric comorbidity among children with gender identity disorder. J Am Acad Child Adolesc Psychiatry 2007;46(10): 1307–14.

11. Massachusetts Department of Education. Massachusetts Youth Risk Behavior Survey. Malden (MA): Massachusetts Department of Education; 2009.

12. Gay Lesbian Straight Educators Network. The 2009 National School Climate Survey: Executive summary. New York (NY): Gay Lesbian Straight Educators Network; 2009. Available at: http://www.glsen.org. Accessed July 14, 2011.

13. Toomey RB, Ryan C, Diaz RM, et al. Gender-nonconforming lesbian, gay, bisexual, and transgender youth: school victimization and young adult psychosocial adjustment. Dev Psychol 2010;46(6):1580–9.

14. Zhao Y, Montoro R, Igartua K, et al. Suicidal ideation and attempt among adolescents reporting "unsure" sexual identity or heterosexual identity plus same-sex attraction or behavior: forgotten groups? J Am Acad Child Adolesc Psychiatry 2010;49(2):104–13.

15. Townsend MH, Wallick MM, Pleak RR, et al. Gay and lesbian issues in child and adolescent psychiatry training as reported by training directors. J Am Acad Child Adolesc Psychiatry 1997;36(6):764–8.

16. Kitts RL. Barriers to optimal care between physicians and lesbian, gay, bisexual, transgender, and questioning adolescent patients. J Homosex 2010;57(6):730–47.

17. Coker TR, Austin SB, Schuster MA. Health and healthcare for lesbian, gay, bisexual, and transgender youth: reducing disparities through research, education, and practice. J Adolesc Health 2009;45(3):213–5.

18. Tamas RL, Miller KH, Martin LJ, et al. Addressing patient sexual orientation in the undergraduate medical education curriculum. Acad Psychiatry 2010;34(5):342–5.

19. Delemarre-van de Waal HA, Peggy Cohen-Kettenis. Clinical management of gender identity disorder in adolescents: A protocol on psychological and paediatric endocrinology aspects. Eur J Endocrinol 2006;155:S1131–7.

20. Spack NP, Edwards-Leeper L. Transgendered youth. In: Fisher M, editor. Textbook of adolescent health care. Elk Grove Village (IL): American Academy of Pediatrics; 2011.

21. Zucker KJ, Bradley SJ, Owen-Anderson A, et al. Puberty-blocking hormonal therapy for adolescents with gender identity disorder: a descriptive clinical study. J Gay Lesbian Mental Health 2011;15(1):58–82.

22. Adolescent Gender Identity Research Group (AGIR). Meeting to develop a consortium of institutions that would form the AGIR-Developing a standard approach to the evaluation of Transgender adolescents held at VUMC. Amsterdam, (Netherlands), May 2007.

23. Zucker KJ, Mitchell JN, Bradley SJ, et al. The Recalled Gender Identity/Gender Role Questionnaire: psychometric properties. Sex Roles 2006;54:469–83.

24. Lindgren TW, Pauly IB. A body image scale for evaluating transsexuals. Arch Sex Behav 1975;4(6):639–56.
25. Deogracias JJ, Johnson LL, Meyer-Bahlburg HF, et al. The gender identity/gender dysphoria questionnaire for adolescents and adults. J Sex Res 2007;44(4):370–9.
26. Cohen-Kettenis PT, van Goozen SH. Sex reassignment of adolescent transsexuals: a follow-up study. J Am Acad Child Adolesc Psychiatry 1997;36(2):263–71.
27. Achenbach TM. Integrative guide to the 1991 CBCL/4-18, YSR, and TRF profiles. Burlington (VT): University of Vermont, Department of Psychology; 1991.
28. Kovacs M. The Children's Depression, Inventory (CDI). Psychopharmacol Bull 1985; 21(4):995–8.
29. Reynolds CR, Richmond BO. Factor structure and construct validity of "what I think and feel": the Revised Children's Manifest Anxiety Scale. J Pers Assess 1979;43(3): 281–3.
30. Conners CK, Barkley RA. Rating scales and checklists for child psychopharmacology. Psychopharmacol Bull 1985;21(4):809–43.
31. Myles BS, Bock SJ, Simpson RL. Asperger Syndrome Diagnostic Scale. Los Angeles: Western Psychological Services; 2001.
32. de Vries AL, Steensma TD, Doreleijers TA, et al. Puberty suppression in adolescents with gender identity disorder: a prospective follow-up study. J Sex Med 2010; 8:2276–83.
33. Wallien MS, Cohen-Kettenis PT. Psychosexual outcome of gender-dysphoric children. J Am Acad Child Adolesc Psychiatry 2008;47(12):1413–23.
34. Cohen-Kettenis PT, Delemarre-van de Waal HA, Gooren LJ. The treatment of adolescent transsexuals: changing insights. J Sex Med 2008;5(8):1892–7.
35. de Vries AL, Noens IL, Cohen-Kettenis PT, et al. Autism spectrum disorders in gender dysphoric children and adolescents. J Autism Dev Disord 2010;40(8):930–6.
36. Di Ceglie D, et al. Children and adolescents referred to a specialist gender identity development service: clinical features and demographic characteristics. Int J Transgend 2002;6(1).
37. Zucker KJ, Bradley SJ, Sanikhani M. Sex differences in referral rates of children with gender identity disorder: some hypotheses. J Abnorm Child Psychol 1997; 25(3):217–27.
38. Gay and Lesbian Medical Association. Guidelines for the care of lesbian, gay, bisexual, and transgender patients. San Francisco (CA): Gay and Lesbian Medical Association; 2006.
39. Radloff L. Center for Epidemiologic Studies Depression Scale (CESD). Applied Psychological Measurement; 1977;1:385–01.
40. Swensen CH, Newton KR. The development of sexual differentiation on the draw-a-person test. J Clin Psychol 1955;11(4):417–9.
41. Bieliauskas VJ. Sexual identification in children's drawings of human figure. J Clin Psychol 1960;16:42–4.
42. Butler RL, Marcuse FL. Sex identification at different ages using the draw-a-person test. J Proj Tech 1959;23:299–302.
43. Zucker KJ. On the "natural history" of gender identity disorder in children. J Am Acad Child Adolesc Psychiatry 2008;47(12):1361–3.
44. Green R. The "sissy boy syndrome" and the development of homosexuality. New Haven (CT): Yale University Press; 1987.
45. Zucker KJ, Bradley SJ. Gender identity disorder and psychosexual problems in children and adolescents. New York: Guilford Press; 1995.
46. Drummond KD, Bradley SJ, Peterson-Badali M, et al. A follow-up study of girls with gender identity disorder. Dev Psychol 2008;44(1):34–45.

47. Zucker KJ. The DSM diagnostic criteria for gender identity disorder in children. Arch Sex Behav 2010;39(2):477–98.
48. Zucker KJ. Reports from the DSM-V Work Group on sexual and gender identity disorders. Arch Sex Behav 2010;39(2):217–20.
49. Meyer-Bahlburg HF. From mental disorder to iatrogenic hypogonadism: dilemmas in conceptualizing gender identity variants as psychiatric conditions. Arch Sex Behav 2010;39(2):461–76.
50. Pleak RR. Ethical issues in diagnosing and treating gender-dysphoric children and adolescents. New York: New York University Press; 1999.
51. Steensma TD, Cohen-Kettenis PT. Gender transitioning before puberty? Arch Sex Behav 2011;40(4):649–50.
52. Rosenberg M. Children with gender identity issues and their parents in individual and group treatment. J Am Acad Child Adolesc Psychiatry 2002;41(5):619–21.
53. Stoddard J, Leibowitz S, Ton H, et al. Improving medical and professional education about gender variant youth and transgender adolescents. Child Adolesc Psychiatr Clin N Am 2011.

Guidelines for Pubertal Suspension and Gender Reassignment for Transgender Adolescents

Wylie C. Hembree, MD

KEYWORDS

- Estrogen • Gender identity disorder
- Gonadotropin releasing hormone agonist
- Puberty Suppression • Testosterone

Over the past 20 years, research studies have established the appropriate age for gender change in adolescents and young adults with persistent gender identity disorder (GID).[1–3] Based on the work of Cohen-Kettenis et al in Amsterdam, it is recommended that children with persistent GID and worsening gender dysphoria begin pubertal suppression at Tanner stage 2 after thorough evaluation by a mental health professional that excludes any psychological disorder causing a gender disorder.[4] This recommendation is part of the Clinical Practice Guideline for the Endocrine Treatment of Transsexual Persons, developed and published by the Endocrine Society and co-sponsored by the European Society of Endocrinology, the European Society of Pediatric Endocrinology, Lawson Wilkins Pediatric Endocrine Society, and the World Professional Association for Transgender Health (WPATH).[5]

The recommendation for pubertal suppression of adolescents with GID is based on 3 observations. First, although 80% to 90% of childhood GID desists by adulthood, GID rarely desists after the onset of pubertal development.[6,7] This conclusion is based on data from a small number of carefully evaluated subjects. In addition, the suppression causes no irreversible or harmful changes in physical development and puberty resumes readily if hormonal suppression is stopped. Second, the onset of the typical physical changes associated with puberty is often associated with worsening of gender dysphoria, distress, and destructive behavior in adolescents with GID.[4] These changes have been reversed by pubertal suppression.[8] Third, hormonal induction of gender-appropriate physical changes is easier and safer when the sex steroids of the adolescent's genetic sex and their physical effects, for example, virilization or breast growth, are not present.[9] The protocol for hormonal treatment of

Department of Medicine, Division of Endocrinology, College of Physicians and Surgeons, Columbia University Medical Center, 101 Central Park West, 1B, New York, NY 10023, USA
E-mail address: wch2@columbia.edu

Child Adolesc Psychiatric Clin N Am 20 (2011) 725–732
doi:10.1016/j.chc.2011.08.004
childpsych.theclinics.com
1056-4993/11/$ – see front matter © 2011 Elsevier Inc. All rights reserved.

adolescents with GID who have undergone pubertal suppression is identical to that used in adolescents with pubertal delay and is associated with few adverse effects.[10]

Historically, attempts to suppress pubertal development of children with precocious puberty that utilized high doses of medroxyprogesterone were associated with only partial suppression and adverse effects owing to its corticoid action.[11] Gonadotropin-releasing hormone (GnRH) is a 10 amino acid peptide synthesized in the hypothalamus. At puberty, GnRH initiates the secretion of pituitary gonadotropins by the pituitary and, thereby, sex hormone secretion by the gonads. The discovery that downregulation of gonadotropin secretion occurred during infusions of GnRH lead to the development of a number of GnRH agonist analogs (GnRHa) that also suppressed gonadotropins.[12] These compounds are now regularly used in a variety of conditions, including, treatment of precocious puberty, endometriosis, disorders of female reproduction, and metastatic prostate cancer.[13] Each use is associated with a very low risk/benefit ratio. Analogs of GnRH with antagonist activity are currently being evaluated for effectiveness in some of these areas,[14] A variety of anti-androgens, anti-estrogens, selective estrogen receptors modulators, selective androgen receptor modulators, and aromatase inhibitors have been suggested as primary and/or adjuvant medications in puberty suppression, although efficacy has been demonstrated in none.

DIAGNOSIS AND DECISION TO TREAT

GID[3] may appear at any age; its manifestations may be subtle or extreme and they are usually well articulated. Behavioral manifestations and ideation vary widely and should be evaluated by a mental health professional. Because GID desists in most, change of gender designation in school or other social circumstances is rarely appropriate during childhood and psychological evaluation is helpful.

A diagnosis of persistent GID is required for consideration of suppression of puberty. This diagnosis should be made by a mental health professional with experience and training in child and adolescent developmental psychopathology.[1,2,4,5,7,8] This is not a diagnosis made by the family of an adolescent, a pediatrician, or an endocrinologist, although efforts to obtain support and understanding of the treatment by the adolescent's family, school, social, and medical team are extremely valuable. The recommendation to begin pubertal suppression must first come from the mental health professional.

The endocrinologist treating the adolescent with GID should confirm the basis upon which the mental health professional has made the recommendation for pubertal suppression.[5] This includes confirmation that the adolescent's GID persists through Tanner stage 2 and exclusion of psychiatric conditions that appear similar to GID or that might interfere with treatment. The Standards of Care of WPATH include six eligibility criteria for adolescents that must be fulfilled and confirmed[15] **(Box 1)**. Adolescents and adults satisfy WPATH readiness criteria for hormone treatment when consolidation of gender identity, improved mental health, and responsible understanding of hormonal treatment are evident.

INITIATION OF GnRH ANALOG TREATMENT

After confirmation of the recommendation for pubertal suppression, the endocrinologist must confirm the good health of the adolescent, explain the reason for the use of GnRH analogs, and, subsequently, sex steroids, review the possible adverse effects,[5] and present the treatment plan and follow-up required. Tanner staging should be confirmed by physical examination and hormone levels. Hormones must be

---

Box 1
Eligibility criteria for puberty suspension, World Professional Association for Transgender Health

1. Fulfillment of DSM and/or ICD-10 criteria for GID or transsexualism;

2. Development to Tanner stage 2 of puberty;

3. Increase in gender dysphoria at the onset of puberty;

4. Psychological and social support;

5. Absence of significant psychologic comorbidity; and

6. Knowledge and understanding of the outcomes of treatment.

Data from Meyer M, Bockting W, Cohen-Kettenis PT, et al. Harry Benjamin International Gender Dysphoria Association's standards of care for gender identity disorder, 6th version. International Journal of Transgenderism 2001;5:1. Available at: http://www.wpath.org/publications_standards.cfm.

---

measured in a clinical laboratory that maintains assays that have sufficient precision and sensitivity to measure the low hormone levels observed in early puberty. Consultation should be maintained with the primary care physician, the mental health professional, and, if psychotropic medications are being given, the prescribing clinician. A complete physical examination provides a good occasion to explain the physical changes anticipated during GnRH analog treatment and when sex hormones are initiated at age 16 years. The physical examination should include assessment of testicular volume and penis width in genetic boys and breast size in genetic girls, and terminal hair distribution in both. Baseline anthropometric data, blood chemistries, bone age, and bone mineral density measurement should be obtained.

It is strongly recommended that initial evaluation should also include a discussion of the effects of treatment on fertility potential and its reversibility. Adolescent or adult endocrinologists should discuss effects of GnRHa and estrogen on sperm production and the option of sperm cryopreservation. In female-to-male (FtM) adolescents, it is helpful to consult a gynecologic reproductive endocrinologist for 3 reasons: (1) To discuss the current status of oocyte cryopreservation techniques available, (2) to discuss possible effects of testosterone treatment on future fertility, and (3) to explain fully the risks and treatment of uterine bleeding during hormone treatment. It is recognized that the age, pubertal stage, sexual knowledge, and behavior of the adolescent and parental consent vary and determine the extent of this discussion. Introduction of these subjects is appropriate at the initiation of treatment, even when the impact on fertility is slight and reversible.

TREATMENT PROTOCOLS
GnRHa

GnRH analog treatment completely suppresses pituitary gonadotropins and, thereby, secretion of the gonadal sex steroids responsible for body changes that have occurred before treatment. The normal adrenal gland produces low levels of testosterone in genetic men and women,[16] the amount of which are insufficient to cause androgenic effects. However, rare genetic abnormalities of adrenal steroid production that result in excess testosterone and, even more rarely, excess estrogen should be excluded. These disorders are usually evident before Tanner stage 2 of puberty.

Chemical modification of the decapeptide, GnRH, has resulted in the marketing of 7 GnRHa used to suppress gonadotropin secretion in a variety of conditions. Studies in adult transsexual persons have utilized treatment with several types of GnRHa.[5] It is likely that any of these 7 GnRHa, properly monitored, will be effective. It is likely that gonadotropin suppression of adolescents with GID will require lower doses of GnRHa than those required for treatment of precocious puberty.

Treatment is usually initiated with monthly injections of depot GnRHa, 3.75 mg. In adolescent boys with GID at Tanner stage 2, the initial dose of GnRHa may be administered at any time. In menstruating girls, GnRHa should first be administered at the onset of menses with an additional dose 2 weeks later to block follicular development that may have occurred after the first injection. Most protocols recommend monthly injections, although careful monitoring of gonadotropin and sex steroid levels may permit increasing the intervals between injections.

Follow-up visits every 3 months should include assessment for adverse effects, anthropometric measurements, measurement of gonadotropin and sex steroid levels, and blood counts. Bone age and bone mineral density may be assessed annually. Rate of growth will slow and bone age will be temporarily delayed. Height stimulation may be considered by the addition of non-virilizing anabolic steroids in FtM adolescents. Final height of male-to-female (MtF) adolescents is usually less than predicted because of early epiphysial closure by estrogens at age 16. Peak bone mass occurs beyond age 20. Adolescents with lipid and glucose metabolism risk factors should be monitored. Adolescent boys with near normal adult levels of testosterone may experience transient hypogonadal symptoms (shorter stature, hot flashes, decreased libido, loss of body hair, reduction in muscle bulk, breast enlargement) during GnRHa treatment. Vasomotor symptoms rarely occur and are treated with tapering dose of progestins.

Sex Steroids

Peer-reviewed, published protocols for puberty suppression in adolescents with persistent GID, followed by administration of the gender appropriate sex steroids, recommend initiation of sex steroid at age 16 years.[5,17] This is largely based on the 20-year Amsterdam studies evaluating the efficacy of initiating treatment at later times.[2,8] In these studies, 140 of 196 adolescents referred were deemed eligible for treatment and, of the 140, 111 received GnRHa suppression. The report on 70 adolescents who received hormone treatment at age 16 demonstrated persistent cross-gender identity and improved psychological functioning in all. The period of puberty suppression before sex steroid treatment is considered to be a diagnostic period during which psychological development improves although GID persists. There are no established criteria for altering the age of steroid administration. Given the constructive outcomes and safety of steroid administration beginning at age 16, it is recommended that earlier treatment be initiated only in exceptional cases decided individually.

Sex steroid administration to hypogonadal adolescents has been demonstrated to be safe and effective. Treatment protocols used for agonadal or hypogonadal adolescents should be utilized at age 16 when eligibility criteria have been fulfilled. These protocols of sex steroid administration will not maintain gonadotropin suppression without continued use of GnRHa.

Daily oral estradiol is recommended for MtF adolescents, based on body size, with increments every 6 months. Intramuscular injection of testosterone esters is recommended for FtM adolescents, given every 2 to 3 weeks. The dose is increased at 6-month intervals. Hormone levels should be measured every 3 months to assess consistent administration of the medication.

Clinical response to sex steroid administration exhibits broad variability. Onset and maximum response have been estimated for adult transsexual steroid treatment.[2]

Breast growth in adult transsexual MtF persons plateaus after approximately 3 years of treatment. Virilization in adult transsexual FtM persons progresses into adulthood, although hirsutism and fat redistribution may begin as early as 6 months. Acne and behavioral changes are common adverse effects of androgen treatment. Breast discomfort, galactorrhea, and increases in prolactin levels may occur with estrogen treatment. Changes in appetite, weight, blood pressure, blood sugar, and lipid levels may occur; most resolve with time.

Undesirable effects

Doses of GnRHa required to suppress sex steroid production in early puberty are rarely associated with side effects. In rare cases, hot flashes may occur, usually do not persist, and can be reduced by low-dose progestins. The growth spurt will not persist or occur, although growth continues. Bone maturation slows, but resumes at the initiation of sex steroid treatment. No studies have evaluated peak bone growth in this protocol. Endocrine modifications may be used when final height may be less than or more than desired. Estrogen-induced hyperprolactinemia is rarely observed.

Although GnRHa in FtM adolescents prevents ovarian estrogen secretion and is probably associated with endometrial atrophy, extraglandular (aromatase) estrogen production from exogenous testosterone may be sufficient to cause vaginal spotting. This can be prevented by oral and/or vaginal progestins.

Adverse effects and metabolic alterations were commonly associated with sex steroid administration to transsexual adults, especially when high doses were used to suppress endogenous steroid production. Adverse effects of exogenous sex steroids rarely occur when GnRHa suppression of endogenous sex steroids is maintained.

Surgery

There are no studies that have evaluated the appropriate timing of surgery as part of the irreversible treatment of adolescent transsexual persons. A threshold of age 18 years is recommended in the WPATH and Endocrine Society guidelines.[5] Mastectomy in FtM adolescents is not recommended before testosterone treatment. Genital surgery may be considered at age 18. GnRHa treatment must be continued along with sex steroids until the gonads have been surgically removed.

CONTROVERSIES
Decision to Treat: Puberty Suppression

Treatment of adolescents with GID is not recommended before Tanner stage 2 of puberty. Only mental health professionals experienced both in the evaluation and management of children and adolescents with GID and trained in child and adolescent developmental psychopathology should make the recommendation to suppress puberty.[5] Adolescents treated with suppression of puberty, followed by sex steroid replacement, maintain their GID and demonstrate improved psychological function.[8] This is in contrast to children with GID not treated at puberty and evaluated in their 20s: GID desists in 80% to 90%.[4,7] Thus, the current standards for evaluation seem to select adolescents whose GID persists and they benefit from puberty suppression.

The success of this protocol depends on the evaluation made by the mental health professional who selects the adolescents who are eligible for puberty suppression and makes the referral to an endocrinologist. Specific appropriate selection criteria have not been published. These criteria can only be established by analysis of a large follow-up study, using a confidential international database in which the details of the evaluation, treatment, and outcome are analyzed. This approach has been used successfully to evaluate outcomes of treatment protocols in virtually every other field of medicine.

Sex Steroid Treatment Before Age 16

Commonly, once treatment for a transition to the appropriate gender is agreed on, sex steroid treatment, with its physical, partially reversible body changes may seem desirable to some earlier than age 16. The Amsterdam group considers the time between Tanner stage 2 and age 16 years as a diagnostic period during which the persistence of the GID becomes more likely, a time for psychological development regarding GID and 16 years old an age when adolescents are much more capable of making partially irreversible changes and the gender role change.

Anecdotal experience with sex steroid treatment earlier than age 16 is widely discussed in the absence of outcome assessment. It is recommended that contact with the mental health professional recommending puberty suppression be continued throughout pubertal suppression to insure continued improvement in management of dysphoria and the complexity of the real-life experience.[15] Together, the mental health professional and the endocrinologist must cautiously assess not only the apparent benefits of early sex steroid treatment, but also the potential harm associated with waiting until age 16 for a particular adolescent.

Fertility Considerations

MtF transsexual adults, before gender transition, may cryopreserve sperm for possible future fertility.[5] FtM transsexual adults rarely have had gonadotropin-induced pregnancy. It is recommended that potential for pregnancy be discussed before sex steroid treatment during endocrine transition. For Tanner stage 2 adolescents with GID, this discussion is more difficult and the options available are limited. However, it is recommended that the mental health professional and endocrinologist initiate the discussion when describing GnRHa blockade, with review of available options again before sex steroid administration.

FUTURE GENITAL SURGERY IN MTF ADOLESCENTS

The skin of the penis and scrotum are used in the construction of a vagina and labia during genital surgery for transsexual women (MtF).[5] The amount of male genital tissue available at Tanner stage 2 is limited and may alter the techniques required for genital reconstruction at age 18. Surgeons have published good results in adolescents following puberty suppression and estrogen administration at age 16.[18]

SUMMARY

The recommendation that pubertal suppression at Tanner stage 2 be considered in adolescents with persistent GID is based on the increase in gender dysphoria and harmful behavior if not treated, the improved psychological functioning during suppression, no change of mind in terms of gender identity, and, in a smaller number who completed sex steroid treatment and surgery, disappearance of dysphoria regarding gender.[18] The ease and safety of long-term GnRHa administration and of hormone replacement protocols in (medication-induced) hypogonadism greatly simplify the endocrine aspect of gender transition. This is in contrast to the adverse effects noted in treatment of transsexual adults in whom endogenous sex steroids are not suppressed.[19,20] Issues related to the achievement of adult height, the timing of initiating sex steroid treatment, future fertility options, preventing uterine bleeding, and required modifications of genital surgery remain areas of concern and further improvement. Concerns have been raised about altering neuropsychological development during cessation of puberty and reinitiation of puberty by the sex steroid opposite those determined by genetic sex.[21] These concerns await resolution in future studies by developmental psychologists and cognitive neuroscientists. In the meantime, thoughtful and careful collaborative assessment and treatment of dysphoric adolescents with persistent GID will resolve these concerns and deepen our understanding of gender development.

REFERENCES

1. Cohen-Kettenis PT, Delemarre-van de Waal HA, Gooren LJ. The treatment of adolescent transsexuals: changing insights. J Sex Med 2008;5:1892–7.
2. Cohen-Kettenis PT, van Goozen SH. Sex reassignment of adolescent transsexuals: a follow-up study. J Am Acad Child Adolesc Psychiatry 1997;36:263–71.
3. American Psychiatric Association (APA). Diagnostic and statistical manual of mental disorders. 4th edition. Washington (DC): Author; 2000.
4. Delemarre-Van de Waal HA, Cohen-Kettenis PT. Clinical Management of gender identity disorder in adolescents: a protocol on psychological and paediatric endocrinology aspects. Eur J Endocrinol 2006;155(Suppl 1):S131–7.
5. Hembree WC, Cohen-Kettenis PT, Delemarre-van de Waal HA, et al. Endocrine treatment of transsexual persons: an Endocrine Society clinical practice guideline. J Clin Endocrinol Metab 2009;94:3132–54.
6. Drummond KD, Bradley SJ, Peterson-Bidali M, et al. A follow-up study of girls with gender identity disorder. Dev Psychol 2008;44:34–45.
7. Zucker KJ. Gender identity disorder in children and adolescents. Annu Rev Clin Psychol 2005;1:467–92.
8. de Vries ALC, Steensma TD, Doreleijers TAH, et al. Puberty suppression in adolescents with gender identity disorder: a prospective follow-up study. J Sex Med 2011;8:2276–83.
9. Delemarre EM, Felius B, Delemarre-van de Waal HA. Inducing puberty. Eur J Endocrinol 2008;159:S9–S15.
10. DiVasta AD, Gordon CM. Hormone replacement therapy for the adolescent patient. Ann N Y Acad Sci 2008;1135:204–11.
11. Sadaghi-Nejad A, Kaplan SL, Grumbach MM. The effect of medroxyprogesterone acetate on adrenocortical function in children with precocious puberty. J Pediatr 1971;78:616–24.
12. Jewelewicz R, Dyrenfurth I, Ferin M, et al. Gonadotropin, estrogen and progesterone response to long term gonadotropin-releasing hormone infusion at various stages of the menstrual cycle. J Clin Endocrinol Metab 1977;45:662–7.
13. Plosker GL, Brogden RN. Leuprorelin: a review of its pharmacology and therapeutic use in prostate cancer, endometriosis and other sex hormone-related disorders. Drugs 1994;48:930–67.
14. Bukulmez O. Biochemistry, molecular biology and cell biology of gonadotropin-releasing hormone antagonists. Curr Opin Obstet Gynecol 2011;23:238–44.
15. Meyer M, Bockting W, Cohen-Kettenis PT, et al. Harry Benjamin International Gender Dysphoria Association's standards of care for gender identity disorder, 6th version. International Journal of Transgenderism 2001;5:1. Available at: http://www.wpath.org/publications standards.cfm. Accessed August 18, 2011.
16. Bardin CW, Hembree WC, Lipsett MB. Suppression of testosterone and androstenedione production rates with dexamethasone in women with idiopathic hirsutism and polycystic ovaries. J Clin Endocrinol Metab 1968;28:1300–6.

17. Olsen J, Forbes C, Belzer M. Management of the transgender adolescent. Arch Pediatr Adolesc Med 2011;165:17117–6.
18. Kreukels BPC, Cohen-Kettenis PT. Puberty suppression in gender identity disorder: the Amsterdam experience. Nature Rev Endocrinol 2011;7:466–72.
19. Asscheman H, Giltay R, Megens AJ, et al. A long-term follow-up study of mortality in transsexuals receiving treatment with cross-sex steroids. Eur J Endocrinol 2011;164: 635–42.
20. Gooren LJ. Care of transsexual persons. N Engl J Med 2011;364:1251–7.
21. Houk CP, Lee PA. The diagnosis and care of transsexual children and adolescents: a pediatric endocrinologist perspective. J Pediatr Endocrinol Metab 200619:103–9.

A Therapeutic Group for Parents of Transgender Adolescents

Edgardo J. Menvielle, MD, MSHS[a,b,]*, Leslie A. Rodnan, MD[a]

KEYWORDS

- Transgender • Gender variant • Parents
- Therapeutic group • Psychotherapy • Transsexual

Therapy for transgender, transsexual, and gender variant persons has traditionally assisted individuals in the process of adjusting to their newly adopted gender role. Increasingly, younger gender variant patients, teens and preteens, present to the clinical consultation raising the need to develop therapeutic interventions that better address the psychosocial needs of minors. The Gender and Sexuality Development Program at Children's National Medical Center (CNMC) in Washington, DC (http://www.childrensnational.org/gendervariance), provides outpatient psychosocial evaluations and therapeutic services for children, adolescents, and their families. The program focuses on addressing the psychosocial needs related to behaviors considered at variance with generally accepted gender roles, gender identity and sexual identity issues, and co-occurring mental health disorders among children and teens whose gender presentations vary from the sanctioned norm. An open-ended group intervention for parents is described, including its format, goals, group composition, and common topics discussed.

THE TRANSGENDER AND GENDER VARIANT TEEN

Gender identity disorder (GID)[1] is a psychiatric diagnosis that applies to persons whose gender identity is different from their assigned gender. The patient experiences a strong and persistent cross-gender identification, discomfort with his or her sex or a sense of inappropriateness in the gender role of that sex, a preoccupation with getting rid of primary and secondary sex characteristics, and significant distress or impairment in social, occupational, or other areas of functioning. Gender dysphoria,

The authors have nothing to disclose.

[a] George Washington University, Washington, DC, USA

[b] Department of Psychiatry, Children's National Medical Center, 111 Michigan Avenue, NW, Washington, DC 20010, USA

* Corresponding author. Department of Psychiatry, Children's National Medical Center, 111 Michigan Avenue, NW, Washington, DC 20010.

E-mail address: EMENVIEL@cnmc.org

Child Adolesc Psychiatric Clin N Am 20 (2011) 733–743

doi:10.1016/j.chc.2011.08.002

childpsych.theclinics.com

which includes discomfort with gender role and a wish of getting rid of natal/pubertal sexual characteristics and acquiring the sexual characteristics of the other gender, may propel an individual to pursue gender reassignment through cross-sex hormones and surgeries. GID is a psychiatric diagnosis that, by definition, emphasizes functional deficits and distress. The term *transgender* is an identity term that refers to the same individuals who are included in the GID category, or at least those who pursue or wish to pursue gender transition. The connotation of the term is a claimed identity and the term does not signal functional deficits or distress. Generally speaking, transgender persons, including adolescents, prefer the term *transgender, transsexual*, or *trans* to describe their experience and do not consider themselves afflicted by a mental disorder, instead viewing their problem as somatic in nature: a body that does not match their sense of self, or a gender role assigned to them based on their biological sex that feels inappropriate or unviable. The main element of the treatment of GID is somatic: helping the patient to achieve his or her desired primary and secondary sexual characteristics through hormonal, surgical, and other auxiliary interventions.[2]

The goal of gender transition among adults and adolescents encompasses the socially successful adoption of the desired gender role including gender-typed appearance and behaviors such as style of clothing and grooming, name, and pronoun use. The therapeutic interventions that may be part of transitioning include cross-sex hormones and other somatic methods to feminize or masculinize the body, surgical interventions of genitals and breasts (eg, construction of a male chest, breast implants, facial feminization), and speech and voice retraining. Depending on the individual characteristics, needs, and preferences, a person may pursue some or all of the elements described.

THE ROLE OF THE CLINICIAN

The role of the clinician is to conduct a comprehensive diagnostic assessment to confirm the diagnosis and assess the conditions that might facilitate, impede, or complicate transition, as well as assisting the person through therapeutic guidance and support. In the case of mature adolescents (age 16 and older) and young adults, surgery is typically postponed until several conditions are met: the patient has reached legal adulthood (18 years old), has achieved a satisfying transition of social role, has had a prolonged course of cross-gender hormones, and is cleared by an experienced mental health professional.[3]

Adolescents undergoing gender transition have to re-work their relationships with parents, siblings, and friends and may also face interpersonal stress and losses, peer bullying and harassment,[4] and sometimes discriminatory restrictions in the use of public accommodations. Levels of depression and suicidal ideation and behavior among transgender persons significantly higher than those of the general population have been reported.[5] Family support has been reported as a psychosocial protective factor for sexual minority youth.[6]

The biggest challenge for teenagers is often related to their parents. In the case of teens who have had a history of childhood gender variance, parents may have, to some extent, prepared themselves for the possibility that their child may be transgender, although the child coming out as transgender often precipitates a crisis within the family. For teens who announce a desire for gender transition without having had a history of childhood gender variance, the crisis may be compounded by the lack of parent's preparation leading to shock and disbelief.[7] Groups for parents have been reported to provide a useful auxiliary intervention for transgender teens.[8]

THE GENDER AND SEXUALITY DEVELOPMENT PROGRAM

At the CNMC's Gender and Sexuality Development Program, patients and parents are evaluated in an initial 120-minute interactive clinical interview that includes the teenager and the parent(s).[9,10] Parents and teens are interviewed together, typically at the start and the end of the assessment session, as well as separately. Standard clinical assessment tools such as the Child Behavior Checklist Youth Self-Report (CBCL-YSR)[11] and Gender Identity Questionnaire[12] supplement the interview.

The clinical interview covers a detailed assessment of gender identity history, sexual behaviors and orientation, and family, peer, and romantic relationships. The presence or absence of concurrent psychopathology, including depression, anxiety, and history of and potential for suicidal behavior, is assessed. Delusional thinking and marked cognitive impairment need to be ruled out.

Social-cognitive difficulties including Asperger and autism disorders and traits, if present, require special consideration. Studies suggest that patients with these conditions may be overrepresented among patients seeking care at specialized gender clinics.[13] The presence of clinically significant sociocognitive problems typically leads to a recommendation for a specialized neuropsychological assessment to inform recommendations for gender transition and to determine the need for concurrent therapy to target the patient's ability to cope with social and occupational demands. A clinical vignette illustrates this point.

> A 16-year-old biological male presented to the gender clinic requesting estrogen treatment. He had never presented socially in a female role, and his overall appearance and grooming were substandard. He had made no serious attempt to explore his feelings while presenting as female. The teen was academically successful but had significant problems with social relationships for all his life. He had never had a mental health assessment. An evaluation by a neuropsychologist supported the diagnosis of Asperger's disorder and individual therapy was started. The teen was originally insistent about initiating hormone therapy to his therapist and a few weeks into therapy was referred back to our group for transgender teens while continuing individual therapy. After a few group sessions, the patient came to the realization, in the individual sessions, that he was fantasizing that gender transition could offer him relief because he was not happy with his life. The patient eventually came to the conclusion that he did not want to be a woman but rather that he was unhappy with his life and that he fantasized gender transition would make him a happier person. The patient left the group and continued individual therapy. Whether the patient reached a permanent resolution of his gender dysphoria, or whether the patient's shift was temporary, is unclear.

ASSESSMENT PROCESS

In the assessment session, we discuss with the youth and the parents the process of transition, the possible ways that transition may occur, with and without the use of hormones and surgery. Potential side effects of hormones, including reproductive implications, are discussed.

Parents typically want to have a confirmation that the teenager's thoughts and feelings are real and that gender transition is necessary for the patient's well-being. Many parents arrive to the assessment stressed, worried about the potential health, social, and occupational implications of undergoing social transition, and sometimes wishing that the patient would reconsider or delay transition.

Parents are sometimes bothered by the vagueness of the diagnosis, which is largely based on the subjective experience and report of the patient. Once the patient is transitioning gender role, parents have to make decisions about how to handle their child's transition vis-à-vis the patient's siblings, extended family, and friends. These issues may begin to be addressed in the assessment session and serve as the basis for recommending participation in our parent group.

EXPECTATIONS FOR TREATMENT

Many youths arrive to the assessment with a wish to start hormones. This occurs both with individuals who have started transitioning socially (sometimes they are already presenting all the time as their affirmed gender) and others whose social transition is incipient. We advise that the teen attend the group a minimum of 3 to 6 months for our team to get to know the patient and his or her family before any final decisions about hormones are made. The group is open-ended, affording the patient the possibility of long-term participation. Referrals for hormone therapy typically occur no sooner than after 3 months of group attendance, although this period may be longer depending on various clinical considerations.

Vignette 1

A 15-year-old Latino biological male had a childhood history of strong preferences for female friends, wearing female clothing and makeup, and making statements about wanting to be a girl. From an early age, the patient showed no interests in team sports or in typically masculine pursuits, despite the father's great efforts to expose him to a variety of sports and martial arts. The parents at some point learned from a babysitter that the patient liked to play with dolls. The teen rarely socialized with other boys, developing friendships exclusively with girls, which is the case to this day. The patient endorsed feeling of being "a mix" of boy and girl, with a 70:30 girl/boy proportion. The teen has always been conscious of his/her parents' disapproval for his/her interests and has made considerable efforts to keep them private. S/he has experimented with makeup since elementary school (at school, so as not to be seen by parents) and female clothing (s/he owns some garments that keeps in private at home). S/he has ventured out dressed as and made up as female successfully and feels "more comfortable" when s/he presents socially as a girl. S/he bleaches and shaves facial hair although s/he appears to have minimal facial hair growth. When going through puberty, the patient hated his "growth" and the appearance of body and facial hair. S/he wants to transition fully to the female gender and undergo surgery to have female genitalia. S/he anticipates that s/he will go through this transition in his 20s. The patient feels exclusively attracted to males as potential sexual and romantic partners but does not endorse having been sexually active.

The patient comes across as a shy teen, soft spoken and somewhat hesitant to answer questions. S/he has an IEP (individualized educational plan) in place, with a history of academic difficulties. S/he also endorses episodes of mild-moderate depression, isolating him/herself socially as a result of his/her feelings and the constraints s/he feels bound by. S/he endorses having had fleeting suicidal thoughts but denies any attempt or plan, past and present.

The patient's parents appear very concerned and embarrassed about the possibility that s/he might cross-dress. The father regards this behavior as a lack of self-respect, and it appears that the opinion of extended family members and their likely disapproval of the child's cross-dressing weigh heavily on their minds.

Vignette 2

A 15-year-old African American biological female has always identified him/herself as a boy. The first memory that the mother recalled was when the child was 3 years old and s/he wanted a dump truck for Christmas. S/he only wanted the truck and had no interest in dolls. As long as s/he has been able to express him/herself, s/he only wanted to shop for clothes in the boys' department. Not long before the clinical consultation, the patient told the mother that s/he is transgender and that s/he feels like a boy. About a month prior, s/he approached the mother and told her that s/he feels like a boy trapped in a female body. The mother was initially somewhat surprised/confused by this revelation as she had thought that the patient may be lesbian: "I did not know what transgender was."

The patient reported that there was no question in his mind that he is a boy except, for his body. He expressed that the chance of his feelings/identity changing in the future was "about 0." The patient reported that he always thought of himself as a boy, but he had not given much thought to his female body until he began developing breasts and had the onset of menses. Both of these developments were very stressful to him. The patient had suicidal ideation at times around body issues, but he did not act on them or made a concrete plan. At the time of the assessment, he wished he could have surgery to remove his breasts as soon as possible and to be able to wear just trunks for swimming again. The patient reported binding his chest using a sports bra and layered baggy clothing to further hide his chest contour.

By the time of the assessment, the patient had told a female friend about his male gender identity. His friend responded positively and encouragingly. He was afraid to tell other people, because he was afraid of being rejected; this included his father (the parents had been divorced for about 12 years) and his school counselor. The patient was also afraid of coming out in school, and he was hoping that the family would move to another state to be close to her mother's family where he could start anew in a school presenting as a boy.

The patient was often mistaken for a boy by strangers, although strangers responded to him as a female sometimes, too. He enjoys being called a boy or young man, and he resents when a friend or acquaintance corrects a newly met acquaintance who assumes that the patient is a biological boy.

Vignette 3

A 17-year-old socially transitioned female-to-male (FTM) transgender teen presented with his parents for an assessment and a referral to hormone therapy. At the time of the appointment, the patient had already been presenting socially as male for several months. He (as she was known prior to transitioning gender) used a male name with co-workers and other persons who he met anew without problems. He had a history of preferring typically masculine play and pursuits since an early age and was considered a tomboy in childhood, developing friendships primarily with male peers and praying not to grow breasts. In middle childhood she (as she was known prior to transitioning gender) once stated, in a Girl Scout meeting, that she would like to be "a man" when she grew up, but otherwise she did not verbally affirm a male identity. The patient was considered a well-adjusted and bright child who excelled in academics and was accepted as a tomboy. Starting in middle school, and following a family move to another part of the country, the patient began struggling with depression and anxiety. She had a brief period in which she tried to dress and groom herself in a feminine manner, but she soon reverted back to a masculine presentation. She became increasingly withdrawn; she lost interest in friends, but still did exceptionally well in school. Social anxiety, present since puberty, became more intense through middle school. In high school the patient became more despondent and agitated; she engaged in repetitive superficial cutting and had suicidal thoughts. As the patient's function deteriorated further, she switched schools several times because of extreme unhappiness with the schools. She was hospitalized in an acute facility and received several months of treatment in a residential facility. Once the patient was stabilized and back at home, he came out to his parents as trans, decided not to re-enroll in school and to pursue a GED (general education diploma) instead, and took an entry-level job in retail. At that point, the patient was functioning well occupationally and within the family but had severed most past peer friendships. At the time the patient was evaluated, his parents had become better informed about transgender issues and were becoming increasingly supportive of the patient presenting as a male at work and public spaces. However, they were also struggling emotionally and with making adjustments within the family such as name and pronoun use. The parents wanted to consult our clinic for a professional confirmation of the patient's transgender identity and to obtain guidance for themselves and their child to handle social challenges, within and outside the family, associated with gender transition. At that time, the child was experiencing significant joy and affirmation from his male presentation and recognition in his job, and he was wishing that his parents would adopt his chosen name and pronoun. He was hoping to start treatment with testosterone in the near future. The patient, who had been seeing a psychotherapist for some time, accepted the internal referral to our group for trans-identified and gender-queer identified youth. The patient had a mostly negative impression of the first group session he attended, but he was encouraged to "stick to it" and soon he became an engaged and productive member of the group.

TEENS AND PARENT GROUPS

At the time of writing this article, the group for adolescents has been meeting for over 2 years and is facilitated by the first author (E.J.M.). The parent group was added as a simultaneous group run by the second author (L.A.R.) together with a second clinician. The age range of teens at the time they joined the group was 13 to 21 years with a median age of 16 years. Of the 23 families (14 FTM and 9 male-to-female [MTF] teens) referred to the group, 19 participated in at least three sessions; one mother and father couple declined ongoing involvement in the parent group while their child attended the teen group; one single parent and child did not come to the group and did not return our calls; and two families came only once and did not return.

Some of groups' therapeutic goals overlap with the goals of individual psychotherapy and include providing an extension of the clinical evaluation, as important aspects of the teens or the parents may have not been observed in the assessment interview. Some other goals are unique to the group modality and include the possibility of observing the patient and the parents interacting with others; providing a social milieu of peers sharing similar experiences and concerns; providing peer support that serves to validate feelings; receiving emotional support and encouragement; and offering instrumental support to others.

Structure of the Parent Group

The sessions are minimally structured, starting with introductions and a few words by each parent about their child including name, age, and a brief description of current status or point of transition. The discussion starts with a parent who volunteers to discuss a point he or she wishes to make or a question for the group.

The group enrolls members on a continuous basis. New members may be initially hesitant to participate while others are very active at first attendance and seem eager to share their experiences, feeling a cathartic relief to be able to discuss their experiences openly and without fear of judgment. It is common, particularly on the first session, for parents to be overtaken with emotion and cry.

Process of the Parent Group

Reactions to the child's coming out and diagnosis

Many parents report that they had no idea about their child's transgender identity until the child communicated it directly to them, as they did not observe gender nonconformity in their child when he or she was younger. Fewer parents had some inkling due to early gender nonconformity, but typically they suspected that their child might at some point identify as lesbian or gay. One father and mother couple reported being shocked to learn that their son felt himself to be female and reportedly had felt so for many years. The father had enjoyed many years acting as scout leader for his son's troup, participating in many camping trips, etc. He claimed to have had no idea at all that there was a gender issue with his child. These parents are regular participants in the group, and while mother's work sometimes prevents her attendance, the father rarely misses a session and is always very engaged and vocal. He often uses humor, although he also sometimes cries. He always expresses loving his child fiercely and feeling a strong desire to protect her from the disapproval, discrimination, and hostility that she may face in society.

Many parents had previously been unfamiliar with the diagnosis of GID or with transgender identity and none have had any personal acquaintance with a transgender person. Most parents initially question whether their child has this diagnosis and wonder if the child is actually going through a phase and/or is being influenced by a social fad or trend, or that this represents adolescent exploration. Over the course of a few months, most parents come to accept the diagnosis.

Although many parents initially have difficultly assimilating the diagnosis, occasionally parents are quick to accept the diagnosis. These are typically parents who see themselves as active problem solvers and avail themselves of every resource that they can find in their community (eg, community meetings for families of transgender persons held by Parents, Families and Friends of Lesbians and Gays [PFLAG]; www.pflag.org), do extensive research on the topic, and tend to move quickly to share this information with other family members and friends (eg, sending out a newsletter). For parents whose children exhibited distress and/or symptoms of psychopathology (depression, self-cutting, anxiety, etc) prior to coming out, knowing what is causing their child's distress finally provides significant relief and a positive sense of closure. On the other hand, some parents worry that the child's newfound sense of peace following coming out and in the early stages of treatment may represent a short-lived honeymoon period that will likely be followed by unhappiness if they experience discrimination, social rejection, and/or disappointments.

"Getting it"

Many parents, like the population in general, initially express that they find relating to the idea of a person wanting to change their gender and sexual characteristics difficult to assimilate. Therefore, appreciating the intensity of feelings and the desperation that some patients experience, is not always grasped. On the other hand, parents often have or develop the meta-cognition acknowledging their difficulty in relating to this, which may allow them to suspend judgment and move toward an increasingly empathic understanding of the patient's predicament. The group process can facilitate this work. For some parents, a change in stance may come suddenly as a sort of revelation or "eureka" moment; for others the change is slow and gradual. A back-and-forth progress, oscillating from understanding and not understanding, is also commonly observed. The group therapist or facilitator has the task of reminding the parents that the feelings of the patient are real and likely permanent. The subjective experience of the patient is not compatible with weighing factors in favor and against transition just as a rational choice. Instead, patients feel that they have almost no choice, or that their choice is restricted to choosing between a guaranteed very low quality life and the possibility of a more fulfilling life.

Coming out to relatives and friends

Anxiety about deciding what to tell and how to tell members of the extended family, and sometimes even close family members, tends to relate to how supportive or tolerant the family is perceived to be and the degree of prior closeness. Families who anticipate more rejection tend to also have more difficulty coming to grips with the permanence of the diagnosis, perhaps because maintaining options open puts off the need to confront potentially hostile relatives.

Reaction to perceived losses

Loss and grief narratives are frequently expressed by group members including the loss of the son or daughter they expected to continue having, and the loss of gender normative hopes, dreams, and expectations for their child's future. Some mourn the loss of a family tradition or aspect of their relationship. The father of an MTF teen mourned the many years of Boy Scout activities he had shared with his son. The mother of an FTM teen expressed sadness in these terms: "She was my only daughter and I was the only daughter of my mother, who was the only daughter of my grandmother."

An almost universal experience for these parents is giving up anticipated stability that parents ordinarily expect to have as their child moves into late teenage years. Instead, they contemplate a more protracted and difficult transition into adulthood, and possibly a longer future with worry and vigilance for their child. Some parents worry about foreclosed reproductive possibilities and feel that their child is not considering the possibility of later in life wanting to have their own biological child (the possibility of banking sperm or eggs is discussed by the group leaders). Worry and fear might eventually subside or vanish when the parents eventually become reassured that the child is on a path to a more or less standard life path that includes school, work, long-term romantic relationships, and/or forming a family. Parents often worry about their child's prospects in finding a loving life partner who accepts a transgender person and about realistic job prospects. These worries may not be new or solely related to the newly disclosed gender identity and gender transition, as for some these same issues were already present and related to preexisting challenges (teens with a lifetime history of social difficulties, anxiety, Asperger/autism traits, depression, etc).

Parents almost universally express anxiety about potential threats to their child's physical and emotional safety, especially during the early transition period when the child may be more easily recognized as transgender or gender variant in public. They are aware of the publicized cases of transgender youth who lost their lives as a result of hate crimes and of the higher statistical chance for depression and suicide among transgender persons. When parents perceive their child as vulnerable to mental health problems, they might reduce their expectations for the child's household and school responsibilities and this can have a detrimental effect. The role of the group therapist or facilitator is to sometimes remind parents that teens often need structure and limits and that, even with generally trusted teens, parents need to use caution. All this is advisable in order to maximize their chances of transitioning successfully into adulthood. Parents sometimes need to be reminded that teens need their support and that this support also includes setting appropriate limits, sometimes requiring curtailing the teen's desires, and often requiring negotiation and compromise.

Transitioning gender at home

Teens and young adults who are living with their parents because they are still in high school, pursuing a GED, or attending a local college, face issues of privacy that in some cases limits the possibility of dressing in the clothes of their choice. This is generally more difficult for MTF teens who may not be able to dress in female attire and grooming in front of both parents, one of the parents, or siblings (or visitors to their home). In our group, most parents have encouraged their child to restrict the cross-dressing to the privacy of their own bedroom or within the home. FTM teens are not affected in the same manner, as they often have been dressing in male attire relatively unimpeded for some time, and in some cases since childhood, since the social reaction to FTM cross-dressing is generally less hostile and may be socially acceptable, such as with tomboys. FTM teens are generally less easily detected in public, especially once they are have been taking testosterone for a few months.

Generally, the parents feel highly stressed in the weeks or months following the disclosure and diagnosis. Some report depression, a sense of confusion and agitation, crying episodes, and social withdrawal. While the child is still living at home, parents feel caught in a dilemma: on one hand, they wish the child not to notice their grief because they do not want to pain their child with a sense of guilt. On the other hand, they often feel that hiding their feelings is a somewhat futile attempt as they are overcome with emotion.

Parents' reactions to the group process

Expressions of gratitude toward the group are common; most parents find that participating in the group as very helpful. The shared experience of emotional toll, confusion, sense of despair, loss, worry, and uncertainty about the future course for their child seems to lessen over time in most cases, although most remain extraordinarily concerned for an anticipated or imagined life of difficulty/pain/isolation/potential for future depression, and so on. There are some parents who come initially and then do not return. Some may feel that group "acceptance" of the diagnosis as well as their child's participating in the concurrent teen group may actually promote a course of action/transition that their child would not otherwise take. One mother found the heart-wrenching story recounted by another mother of her child's struggle with severe depression, social isolation, and chronic suicidal ideation to be so stressful that she did not return for subsequent group sessions though her husband has continued to participate.

SUMMARY

The themes that arise in group interactions among parents of transgender and gender variant teens have much in common with themes that arise during the initial assessment and during parent or family sessions in the context of providing psychotherapy for these patients. The group process, however, affords some distinct advantages. The first one is that themes that might have not come up in the treatment of an individual or a family might be brought up by another group member and be relevant to this family. In other words, a group provides a greater number of relevant topics of discussion, some of which might not be raised by a single individual or single family. Second, a group sanctions topics that might be difficult for a single individual or family to talk about. Listening to the stories of others, in addition to talking, can be very valuable, providing insight and emotional and instrumental support. In a group, parents model for each other acceptance and ways of coping with difficult challenges through pooling their problem solving skills. Comments like "It never occurred to me to talk about it in that way . . . or to do that" are common and reveal the utility of the group process for parents dealing with a very stressful reality.[14–18]

REFERENCES

1. American Psychiatric Association. Diagnostic and statistical manual of mental disorders. 4th edition, text revised. Washington, DC: American Psychiatric Association; 2000.
2. Hill DB, Rozanski C, Carfagnini J, et al. Gender identity disorder in children and adolescents: a critical review. Int J Sexual Health 2007;19:95–122.
3. WPATH (World Professional Association for Transgender Health). The Harry Benjamin International Gender Dysphoria Association's standards of care for gender identity disorders. 6th edition. Available at: http://www.wpath.org/publications_standards.cfm. Accessed August 18, 2011.
4. Pleak RR. Formation of transgender identities in adolescence. J Gay Lesbian Ment Health 2009;13(4):282–91.
5. Clements-Nolle K, Marx R, Katz M. Attempted suicide among transgender persons. J Homosexuality 2006;51(3):53–69.
6. Ryan C, Huebner D, Diaz RM, et al. Family rejection as a predictor of negative health outcomes in white and Latino lesbian, gay, and bisexual young adults. Pediatrics 2009;123(1):346–52.
7. Lev AI. Transgender emergence: therapeutic guidelines for working with gender variant people and their families. New York: Haworth; 2004.
8. DiCeglie D, Thümmel EC. An experience of group work with parents of children and adolescents with gender identity disorder. Clin Child Psychol Psychiatry 2006;11:387–96.
9. Hill DB, Menvielle E, Sica KM, et al. An affirmative intervention for families with gender variant children: parental ratings of child mental health and gender. J Sex Marital Ther 2010;36:6–23.
10. Hill DB, Menvielle E. "You have to give them a place where they feel protected and safe and loved": the views of parents who have gender-variant children and adolescents. J LGBT Youth 2009;6(2–3)6,7.
11. Achenbach TM. Integrative guide to the 1991 CBCL/4-18, YSR, and TRF profiles. Burlington (VT): University of Vermont; 1991.
12. Johnson LL, Bradley SJ, Birkenfeld-Adams AS, et al. A parent-report Gender Identity Questionnaire for Children. Arch Sex Behav 2004;33:105–16.
13. de Vries A, Noens I, Cohen-Kettenis P, et al. Autism spectrum disorders in gender dysphoric children and adolescents. J Autism Dev Disord 2010;40(8):930–6.
14. Menvielle E, Hill DB. An affirmative intervention for families with gender variant children: a process evaluation. J Gay Lesbian Ment Health 2011;15:1–20.
15. Cohen-Kettenis PT, van Goozen SH. Sex reassignment of adolescent transsexuals: a follow-up study. J Am Acad Child Adolesc Psychiatry 1997;36(2):263–71.
16. Hembree WC, Cohen-Kettenis PT, Delemarre-van de Waal HA, et al. Endocrine treatment of transsexual persons: an Endocrine Society Clinical Practice Guideline. J Clin Endocrinol Metab 2009;94(9):3132–54.

17. Smith Y, Van Goozen S, Kuiper A, et al. Sex reassignment: outcomes and predictors of treatment for adolescent and adult transsexuals. Psychol Med 2005;35(1):89–99.
18. Zucker KJ, Cohen-Kettenis PT. Gender identity disorders in children and adolescents. In: Rowland DL, Incrocci L, editors. Handbook of sexual and gender identity disorders. Hoboken (NJ): John Wiley & Sons; 2008. p. 376–422.

Snakes and Snails and Mermaid Tails: Raising a Gender-Variant Son

Tony Kelso, PhD

KEYWORDS

• Gender nonconformity • Gender atypical • Gender stereotypes • Parenting • Support groups

"There's the penis," the sonographer pointed out after we had repeatedly confirmed that we wanted to know the sex of our baby-to-be protruding from Tricia's stomach. Immediately my heart dropped swiftly into my own stomach. For a few moments of slow-motion haze, all the life went out of me. How could it be? Both my wife and I knew we were having a girl. My mom said we were having a girl. Every friend who knew us well said we were having a girl. I wanted a girl.

Sitting in the reception area waiting for Tricia to finish changing her clothes, tears began to edge slowly down my cheeks. Pictures of my childhood flashed before my mind's eye—not just any images, but scenes between my father and me: the time he shouted at me like a wild man through an entire wash cycle because I had splashed through a few puddles on my way home from school. The time he threw me into the bedroom after choking me in the hall, then a few minutes later called me out of the room to ask with a syrupy voice if he had hurt me and finally screamed after I had nodded yes through my tears, "GOOD!" The time, as my mother came to a halt in the driveway to take me swimming after she had vanished for days to escape my father's unending wrath that he slugged her so hard she bit her tongue, oozing her warm blood onto the front seat. The time he verbally attacked me, then 11 years old, for not fighting the divorce my mother had recently filed for. The time, while my parents were separated before the divorce was final, my mom and I checked into a motel for the night because she had received a call from her best friend in Nebraska who said she had just heard from my father, who revealed that he was on his way to murder us. The time I came home after a Pony League baseball game to discover my battered mother shivering and huddled in a corner after my father had broken into the house through the milk shoot to greet her with force. The Sundays after the divorce when he would pick me up, speed 60 miles per hour down the residential street from my house with a crazed expression, stop in a parking lot, then hostilely explain to me how my mother

Department of Mass Communication, Iona College, New Rochelle, NY 10801, USA
E-mail address: AKelso@iona.edu.

Child Adolesc Psychiatric Clin N Am 20 (2011) 745–755
doi:10.1016/j.chc.2011.07.003
1056-4993/11/$ – see front matter © 2011 Elsevier Inc. All rights reserved.

was a pig and a whore who hung out with other pigs and whores. No, I was not prepared to father a son.

Eventually though, before the birth I came to terms with having a baby boy. Once our baby graced our lives, despite my selfishness and my own angry temper, I struggled to become the best parent I could be. There's no doubt I felt the sensation a friend had once said I would when I looked into the eyes of my new baby. "It's like falling in love again," he smiled. Honestly, how could you not love the little fellow? My God, he was cute. And not in that he's-my-baby-so-of-course-he's-cute sort of way. I could tell he was adorable by anybody's standards. Pretty, even.

Later, soon after Aron had learned to walk, I privately gloated over what a progressive parent I was when I bought him a pair of striped girls' platform flip-flops. After all, didn't Aron show fascination for the girls' shoes sitting beside the sandbox while toddling through the playground? Why not get him his own pair? He was only a year old—it didn't mean anything. Nor did I find it alarming to walk through the park with my son as he held a blond-haired doll a friend of Tricia's had just given him because he had noticed it on her shelf and wanted to play with it. Sure I received a few stares from some of the other ambling fathers—but it wasn't my problem if they were closed-minded and couldn't match my liberal propensity to go with the flow. I knew it was just a phase.

***

"Boy, you sure are pretty," I said to Aron, now 3, while he displayed the first dress we had given him. Truth be told, I loathed looking at him in the light violet and flowered gown he was wearing. But I forced myself to pretend and say something positive. Could he tell I was faking? Then again, was I really feigning? Realizing he needed my approval, I was sincere in my fakery. His eyes beamed and his smile lit up the room as he hugged me. Filled with convoluted emotions, I could clearly recognize only one of them—guilt.

The guilt haunted me day after day. Yes I allowed my son to dress like a girl (only at home), to act like a girl, to play with dolls, to draw mermaids, to watch *Angelina Ballerina* on television. But always through gritted teeth. I scolded myself for merely tolerating who he was, for not utterly embracing his gender-nonconforming activity. On top of that, I berated myself for not living up to my convictions. Here I was, a PhD-holding scholar of media, a professor who lectured students in his Race and Gender in Mass Communication courses about the social construction of gender, gender stereotypes, gender fluidity, and the damage that identity biases could evoke. I had read the books. I could quote Judith Butler, a feminist post-structuralist philosopher. Intellectually I understood and adopted the ideas associated with "queer theory." Yet on a visceral level, as much as I strove to make it happen, I could not bring myself to swallow the everyday experience of seeing my son enter our apartment after returning from nursery school and immediately ripping off his clothes in the hallway, running to his bedroom, and putting on his dress and the cap that held in place his "long hair"—a green and white pom-pom that we had brought home after a father-son night at a college basketball game.

The moment of epiphany when Tricia and I suddenly realized our son was definitely "different" occurred the evening Aron's day care center held a graduation ceremony for the 3-year-old children who were moving on to nursery school. As the young girls and boys lined up before us in their shiny white caps and gowns, "Miss D" (the moniker she chose to go by) read off the name of each youngster and said a few words about him or her. Summarizing her general impressions, she delivered a string of predictable capsules. ("Suzi loves to sing," "Nathan is great with Lego," and so on.)

Yet when she came to Aron, the first words out of her mouth were, "Aron, who has a deep appreciation for feminine beauty . . . ." I heard little after that. All the signs swiftly crystallized: The Barbie doll styling head, which our neighbors had given him for Christmas when he was 2, no longer came across as just a novelty. His favorite present that year, for months he carried it around everywhere he went—even halfway around the world to the Philippines when we visited Tricia's family—like a trophy he had earned by decapitating his stunning victim in a barbaric war. It all became clear—the beads he enjoyed holding, the blue wig he donned while walking down the streets of Manhattan, the attraction to everything pink. I remembered the first time I had tried to explain the difference between boys and girls by pointing a few out near our apartment then asking what gender he was, to which he replied, "I'm a boy *and* a girl." These articles, behaviors, and expressions were not a passing fancy. To the contrary, they captured the essence of a little boy who from then on would challenge the lifetime of gender socialization Tricia and I had both received.

***

Before surrendering to the idea he should have a dress, I went through the inevitable stage of denial that entailed trying to find acceptable substitutes for his decidedly feminine yearnings. "Maybe a Ken doll instead of a Barbie," I reasoned to myself. We bought him a slight variation, "Steven," a Ken doll tinted brown to make him African American. He didn't look as obnoxiously wholesome as his white buddy. Yet the toy sat idle or merely watched his girl counterparts prepare for the ball. "What about a Native American outfit?" I rationalized. Maybe all the fancy feathers and bold colors will satisfy him. Perhaps a Chinese, Indian (as in, from the nation of India), or African ensemble—they certainly are more vibrant than our American gray suits. Or if he likes skirts, then why not a Scottish or Irish kilt? I showed him pictures of men in these plaid "dresses." Aron didn't seem interested, as though he could see through my feeble attempt at compromise. No, he didn't want some homely checkered pattern worn by people with hairy legs—he craved the real thing.

***

In a strange way, at least for a while, our son's gender variance brought Tricia and me closer together. In bed before falling asleep, Tricia would often cry, and we would comfort one another about what felt like the loss of our son. For Tricia, the pain involved not wanting to stand out, a way of life tacitly frowned upon by the Filipino culture she had grown up in. For me, it was, well, it was hard to say. For as long as I could remember I had taken pride in my independent spirit, in my never-ending inclination to not go along with the crowd. Nor was Aron's girlishness a threat to my own masculine identity. I wasn't saddled with the need to exude machismo with every utterance and gesture. Yes, I earnestly followed sports. But I also took great pleasure in watching dance, cried at movies, and engaged in long conversations centered on feelings.

Part of what made adapting to the prospect of raising a gender-variant boy so difficult was that Tricia and I had almost no support network. We found little consolation in turning to our neighborhood friends. And the judgment we received wasn't what one might expect. Nobody scolded us for buying our son a toy oven (well, actually, Tricia's mom did mention it in passing once). None of the moms and dads in our social circle took us to task for allowing him to play with Barbies. In short, we weren't chastised for somehow "turning him into a girl" by permitting him to follow his own female-like tastes. Rather, we felt rejected because, in our politically liberal, yuppyish section of Northern Manhattan, people couldn't understand why we were battling to accept having a little "girl-boy" (the designation Aron himself had introduced into our family lexicon). So what if he turns out to be gay? So what if sexual reassignment was a future possibility? He was our kid and it was our duty to love him unconditionally. As if we didn't already know that, thank you very much. As if we weren't trying our best. "So easy for them to say," I often thought. Momentarily looking at somebody else's boy in a fairy outfit might come across as charming to the free-thinking outsider taking delight in witnessing a preschool child subvert gender norms. But it's not so effortless when it's your own boy drifting off to la-la land day after day, week after week, month after month. Instead of resting in the solace of a fellow parent's understanding, confiding in our friends only exacerbated our sense of shame for failing to celebrate our son's unconventional expression. There was that guilt again.

The tension between either being mildly rebuked or having our sense of sadness readily dismissed and pining for empathy almost destroyed a close relationship. I was at our neighbors' apartment a few months after the revelatory episode at our son's day care commencement exercises. (This was the home of the married couple who had, without telling us first, given Aron the Barbie doll styling head, a gesture I had ever since privately resented and deemed unacceptably presumptuous.) Susan and Robert (names changed to protect privacy) had two children of their own, both daughters (naturally, Aron much preferred the company of girls over boys). Aron adored the older kid, who had been born almost exactly one year before him. We trafficked back and forth between our apartments as though we were one big family. Inevitably when Aron was at their place he and the girls would play dress-up, transforming themselves into princesses or other frilly characters. Weeks before though, in an attempt to somehow monitor Aron's atypical gender behavior, we had asked Susan and Robert if they could speak with their daughters about not loaning any of their possessions to him—we had enough hyperfeminine playthings and garments spilling from Aron's toy boxes. We recommended the policy be mutual and that we offer a pseudoexcuse such as, "If you loan something out it might get lost." They accepted our appeal. Yet here was the older girl telling Aron it was okay if he wanted to borrow one of her ornate accessories that rounded out the gaudy outfit—complete with pink dress and high-heeled shoes—he was currently wearing. I turned to Susan and Robert and discretely yet desperately asked if they would remind their daughter about our new rule. During the awkward exchange, however, the scene quickly became contentious.

"It's not our problem if you can't handle a boy in a dress!" Robert shouted.

"You don't understand!" I shot back.

"We don't understand?" Susan screamed. Then she went off on a rage.

"Get out!" Robert yelled as Susan continued howling.

Treasuring their friendship, a day or so later I invited them to meet Tricia and me at a restaurant so we could patch things up. Fortunately we made amends and Aron continues to happily play with the daughters.

***

Our path to learning how to fully appreciate and fruitfully rear a "pink boy" actually began the day after Miss D's illuminating observation at the day care graduation. That morning as soon as I arrived at my office at the college, I combed the books on my shelf filed under gender. Locating one or two key texts, I quickly skimmed through them for insight. Then I turned to the Internet. I didn't have to search long before I uncovered a pamphlet published by the Children's National Medical Center (CNMC) in Washington, DC titled, "If You Are Concerned About Your Child's Gender Behaviors: A Guide for Parents."[1] Yep, that was me. I read on.

By the age of 3 years, most children express an interest in or preference toward activities and behaviors typically associated to their specific gender. . . . However, some children develop in a different way. Some children have interests more typical of the other sex and sometimes want to look and act like the other sex. For example, a 7-year-old boy plays with Barbie dolls and pretends to have long hair and be a princess.

Just like that I recognized my son and, although a wave of sorrow washed over me, I took hope in realizing there was a possible entrance to the road of understanding.

Dialing the number on the back of the brochure, Tricia and I were able to set up a conference call with Catherine Tuerk, RN, one of the co-founders of the CNMC (see Tuerk's article in this volume). "Finally," I thought during the conversation, "a person who identifies with what we're going through—and can truly offer some sound advice."

"Tell your son there are different types of boys. A lot of boys like cars and toy soldiers. But some boys enjoy 'girl' things like dolls and dress-up."

I hung on her words as though she were a spiritual master teaching me how to hear the sound of one hand clapping.

The primary support mechanism that the CNMC provides is an e-mail Listserv through which parents around the country raising gender-variant children can exchange stories and tender bits of wisdom, or at the very least lend a sympathetic ear. About 2 months after Aron's 3-year-old birthday I posted our account. I received an outpouring of encouragement. "I can only speak for myself . . . but I was where you are now. My husband is still learning to be more accepting," one woman wrote. "Based on your thoughtful evolution, Aron will grow up to be a wonderful secure and happy person, I am sure of it!" another chimed in.

Hearing from a father was especially meaningful to me. A man from Utah confided, "Boy, can I relate to your feelings . . . though you are light-years farther along than I was when Ken (name changed to protect privacy) (7) was 3. At that time we still were quite 'mean' to him from lack of understanding. Lots of things we did, and his innocent reaction, just make me cringe and cry now to think about it."

Yet I came to discover that the Listserv was mainly used by parents who had already reconciled any negative feelings they had harbored about nurturing their pink boys and were instead involved in advocating on behalf of their sons and challenging their neighbors, friends, families, and educators to expand their concept of gender. No doubt this was an admirable cause, I recognized. But I simply wasn't ready to join the march when my own emotions were so ambivalent. And because I consistently compared myself to the "enlightened" members of the Listserv who reveled in crafting shrines to Barbie (one parent revealed that her family had actually done this), I could only judge myself even more harshly. The guilt continued to flow.

Tricia's discomfort with the Listserv was greater still. She couldn't cope with hearing about boys who were already apparently transitioning into girls. "Hope your holiday finds you well and at peace with your child's g.v. [gender variant] expression. As a gift to Kirk (name changed to protect privacy), we decided to stop fighting about the dress and allowed one for Christmas mass. We purchased a red satin blouse and a black skirt with red trim," wrote a woman from Indiana. Would Aron eventually want to strike a similar pose? Tricia couldn't endure the image of our son one day soon not only frolicking around in a flowery dress at home but animatedly displaying his clothing from the Target girls' rack at school, in church, and on the playground. Discussion about shifting pronouns, allowing a boy to use the nurse's instead of the boys' or girls' bathroom at school, and a parent searching high and low for a ballet instructor who would allow a son to wear a tutu to class like the girls was more than she could take. Yet even more gut-wrenching for her were the tales of the bullying and the abuse from both peers and blinkered grown-ups that some of the children had to face, incidents that could one day be part of Aron's reality. She stopped reading the posts.

The dangers of straying too far from the tacit Listserv consensus became clear when a gentleman from New Zealand, while introducing himself to the group, betrayed mixed emotions about his son. "We would endeavour to support him to the best of our ability if he indeed turns out to be gender-variant and perhaps even gay, but to be honest, we would much prefer him to be a typical 'straight' boy. Consequently, we would never force him to do gender-typical things that he was really uncomfortable with, but we also do not wish to encourage (the further development of) effeminate behaviour."

A gay parent delivered a faint reproach in his response. "I respect your honesty about your hopes and wishes for Stuart (name changed to protect privacy). But if I may be blunt in a typical American way, I believe that your choice around 'encouragement' is to encourage Stuart either to be himself and happy, or to be someone else and not happy. You didn't do anything to make him this way (witness your two other children) and you aren't going to find any harmless way to change him."

The man from New Zealand clarified what he was looking for. "So the question remains; is our son gender-variant and/or likely to be gay, or not. If he is, why is he missing so many of the key ingredients? If he isn't, does his atypical behaviour constitute some other thing to be 'concerned' about, or are we 'making mountains out of molehills?'"

I knew reaching out to the group to receive a firm diagnosis was misguided. Yet by no means did the New Zealand parent come across as horribly small-minded; to me he seemed like a typical father who for the first time was confronting the fact that his son defied customs he himself had always associated with masculinity. That father deserved a kind word despite not measuring up to the Listserv's general stance on gender variance—indeed, falling short of the mark was all the more reason to render support. Yet what he got was often judgmental in tone. One father was especially critical.

What's painful for us, is that while you are voicing your support, you are also subtly exhibiting signs of not being supportive. It is almost as if you are looking for us to confirm your "diagnosis" so you could seek some form of behavioral therapy to prevent your son from "becoming" gay.

Your son, if he is anything like many of our sons, picks up on your ambivalence; this may be acting as a curb on his expression. He knows that what he wants to be is not acceptable. So you may be confounding the experiment without realizing it . . . .

So there is no "encourage" or "discourage." There's "acceptance," and "lifetime of misery and greatly elevated risk of suicide." That's your choice. Which means you have no choice.

Ouch. Needless to say, the Listserv never again heard the voice from New Zealand—the gentleman had been chased away. I learned that a type of groupthink was at work and that I had better be careful about expressing any tentativeness I had about my son growing up gay or even transgendered.

Yet the Listserv proved useful in other ways. It was a great source for finding out about books and movies that center on gender variance. What's more, in spite of the participants' resistance to other parents who weren't on board (which, of course, I was—I was just having a tough time processing my own inner conflict), they without doubt presented a lot of helpful anecdotes on how they had navigated certain issues that inevitably arise when you are rearing a boy who wishes he could be a girl—from dealing with a bully at school who won't stop teasing your son to what to say when a person at the mall remarks, "Your daughter is so cute." Not to mention it was comforting to merely find out there were other families with boys like Aron.

Probably the best thing to come out of our connection with the CNMC, however, was obtaining the contact information of a psychiatrist in the New York area, Richard R Pleak, MD, who specializes in gender nonconformity in children. Like the parents on the Listserv, Dr Pleak didn't believe in "treating" your son until he suddenly declares a passion for football. Similarly, Dr Pleak's approach involved loving your boy for who he is and allowing him to express his interests: I wouldn't force a "normal" son to stop playing with a safe toy he utterly enjoyed; why would we do so with Aron? Yet one of the qualities we most appreciated about Dr Pleak was that he seemed to convey a more cautious attitude than many of the Listserv parents toward bringing up a gender-variant kid. For example, he advised us not to allow Aron to wear a dress at school—or any other public setting. Instead, he recommended that we provide a safe haven at home for him to slip on a princess crown or design a new outfit for Barbie—not because boys shouldn't do such things, but to shield him from the taunting that would surely result. He was plainly too young to handle it effectively. But what would we say when he asked why he couldn't wear girls' clothes once he exited our door? We decided to tell him that people don't wear costumes outside. After all, although Aron had more in common with girls than his own sex, he had never disputed the fact that he is a biological boy. Ah, the matter was settled.

"But Eddie gets to wear a Superman costume outside," Aron said one day.

Goddamn Eddie. Aron had me—Eddie was indeed allowed to wear the man of steel's tights and cape beyond the home. In fact, Eddie was allowed to appear in his Superman guise *every day*. Apparently his parents were permitting him to work through his superhero phase. But we weren't dealing with a passing stage of development.

"Eddie's family has different rules than our family," I answered. Oh great. How do I explain ethical relativity to a 3-year-old? "Actually, most families have the same rule as us," I added. "But just like there are different types of people in the world, there are different types of families." What a wimpy response. I quickly resorted to changing the subject.

Perhaps the most valuable tactic we acquired through our conversations with Dr Pleak was, as much as possible, to resolve conflicts apart from the realm of gender. If Aron wanted to take his Polly Pockets to the park, rather than warn him with, "Boys shouldn't be seen with dolls," we could go with "Let's leave her home—she's too small and might get lost." If he wanted to paint his nails or put on lipstick we could say, "Makeup isn't for kids. You need to wait until you're older to start using it."

Along with following this general guideline, we also—again, with Dr Pleak's encouragement—made it a point to leave all options open. If we let Aron persistently present as a girl, then what stresses would emerge if he wanted to change back two months from now?

***

"Follow his lead," the people on the Listserv constantly advised. If he wants to be a boy who wears dresses to school, then let him be a boy who wears dresses to school. If he wants to identify full time as a girl, then let him identify full time as a girl.

"Bullshit!" I growled to myself. How could a 3- or 4-year-old kid possibly make such an important decision—particularly on a concern so central to his very identity? Wasn't it our job as parents to make these kinds of weighty choices for him? Should we let him eat ice cream three times a day because he loves that too? Yes, it would be nice, should Aron declare he wishes to dress like a girl full-time, if his teacher and all of the staff at school welcomed his new attire, not a single parent complained, and none of his friends batted an eyelash at the switch. But that's not the real world—nor will it be anytime soon, if ever. Rather than teach Aron how to fit into his environment, should we expect everybody else to accommodate him by magically assuming the latest, most progressive views on gender? I wasn't ready to make Aron a guinea pig and turn him into an activist for GLBT (gay, lesbian, bisexual, transgender) rights. I scoffed at the parents on the Listserv who had already allowed their sons—some as young as 5 or 6—to transition into girls with penises, given them other names, and enrolled them at different schools so their youngsters could start anew with fresh identities. Yes, I'm liberal. But this was child-centered parenting to the extreme. Had these people been sucked in by the ideological trends that stipulate we must masochistically become hyperparents or helicopter parents, eternally striving to meet our children's needs while dying to our own? Surely it's time to put the parental foot down when little Donny insists he now wants to be Daisy.

It took me literally years to modify my stance on this issue and realize that in some cases, loving parents really have no choice but to help their sons convert into daughters. When I heard stories about boys who persistently screamed, "I AM A GIRL!," threw daily tantrums as they slipped on trousers, talked about cutting off their penises or worse yet, killing themselves, but when later were permitted to be girls suddenly seemed happier than they had ever been in their lives, then who was I to judge their parents' decisions? When a young boy's passion to be female trumps any concern about being beat up by a school bully, teased by kids on the playground, or belittled by a teacher in the classroom, then to deny that child's deepest desire would be downright cruel. But what if he wanted to change back later? Well, I contemplated, his mother and father would simply have to cross that hurdle when it came.

Fortunately, Tricia and I have never faced such a quandary. In no way has Aron consistently pointed this far toward the end of the gender-variant spectrum. Still, I often worry—accompanied by those perpetual feelings of guilt—if the reason he has never insisted on crossing over to the other side is because he used to sense, despite me going along with him, my discomfort and even underlying hostility when he played beauty shop with twelve dolls lined in a row or inevitably selected one of the most girly-girl books at Barnes & Noble whenever we asked which one he'd like us to buy. How many times had I made an offhanded comment—its bitterness barely veiled—when all my son wanted to do was have fun with his toys just like the rest of the kids?

***

Besides putting us in touch with Dr Pleak, the Listserv has also led to other indispensible face-to-face interactions. Nearly 2 years ago, on Aron's last day of kindergarten, I picked him up and together we headed by car to Washington, DC, where we attended the group's annual Camp I Am, a weekend retreat for families with gender-variant sons. While the parents visit, share stories, and hear speakers, the boys have the opportunity to meet other boys who gravitate toward pink and can unabashedly be themselves in an accepting environment. The culminating event at the camp is a red-runway fashion show with the boys in drag and parading their wares to the roaring cheers of their parents. Immersed in a land in which gender noncon-formity becomes normal, instead of recoiling at the prospect of my son prancing about as a girl, I found myself in the bathroom before the show frantically helping Aron get ready and look his best in his white dress with striped sleeves, long black boots, and blonde wig, an ensemble Aron himself had designed by piecing together items he already owned with garments he had picked out in the girls' section of a children's clothing store. As he strutted his stuff down the aisle, I earnestly beamed. "That's my boy," I said to myself.

Less than a year after the Camp I Am episode, two parents on the Listserv formed Stepping Stones, a support group in Manhattan for families in the Tri-State area of New York, New Jersey, and Connecticut with either sons or daughters who display atypical gender behavior. (See Wisnowski's article in this volume. – ed.) Today I look forward to the monthly meetings, which are held at a PFLAG (Parents, Families, and Friends of Lesbians and Gays: www.pflag.org) center. After dropping Aron off with a leader who guides the kids in a fun activity in one room, Tricia and I join the rest of the parents in a circle in another room to discuss our issues. By putting faces to the fingers of some of the people on the Listserv I have discovered they aren't all militant activists who graduated from Berkeley or the like and hit the panic button whenever their children swallow a morsel that isn't organic. No, they're just everyday folks encompassing a broad range of personalities and backgrounds (although, I must admit, I have met relatively few people of color among them). Freed from their keyboards and surrounded by actual bodies, the parents at Camp I Am and Stepping Stones are able to let down their guard and say things that probably wouldn't fly on the Listserv.

***

I first noticed that Aron wasn't sporting his dress at home every day about a year after we had first purchased it for him. Tricia's mom was visiting us from the Philippines, and I wondered if he was aware of his grandmother's uneasiness with his gender expression and had thus resolved to remain in his T-shirt and jeans while she stayed in town. (See a discussion of such suppression in the Stoddard and colleagues article in this issue.– ed.) Although my mother-in-law, to her credit, had always—albeit grudgingly—supported our approach, she had nonetheless let loose with the occasional remark that told Aron how she wasn't completely happy about his unconventional manner. Yet when I asked him why he wasn't wearing his favorite garment as often as he used to, he gave a vague answer. That was generally his style. Whenever Tricia or I tried to talk with him about anything relating to gender, he was usually evasive. Then again, to this day Aron tends to be circumspect about almost any personal matter. Of course it probably didn't help that just about every time I attempted to explore the realm of gender with him I came across about as smoothly as a teenage boy breaking up with his girlfriend. I never could phrase things right. Still, it wasn't entirely my fault. Discussing any deep-rooted issue with a person who was in diapers only 2 or 3 years ago is no easy task.

Nonetheless, the telltale sign for me has always been, *Does Aron seem happy?* And, thankfully, the answer all along has been *Yes*. He has never withdrawn from us or his peers, given enduring signals of depression or self-hatred, or indicated that being a boy is unbearable. Sure he has an angry temper, is bull-headed (ie, "spirited," according to the latest politically correct terminology) to the nth degree, and incessantly complains whenever something isn't exactly the way he wants it. But that's just Aron. He'd be the same whether he was a boy or a girl.

The truth is Aron is incredibly vibrant. When he laughs, he does so with every ounce of his being—and transports me to a place of joy in the process. His energy is boundless (we think he has ADHD [attention deficit-hyperactivity disorder], but that's a whole other story). When he walks into a room, he permeates it with his presence.

The kid is so affectionate—yet not in a clingy way—that at times it can be downright annoying. For sure nobody has ever looked at Aron and said, "Boy, is he a miserable kid." So maybe Tricia and I haven't done such a bad job parenting after all.

Today at 7 years old, Aron more or less leads a double life. He still loves fantasizing with his Barbies—although not as obsessively as before. He still prefers playing with girls over boys. He'd still rather draw flowers than guns. Yet he is careful about whom he shares—as he puts it—his "secret," with, which is (again, his words) that he likes "girl things." When he's at school, he keeps his dolls in his bag—or leaves them at home altogether. He picks and chooses which friends to confide in about his class at the School of American Ballet. (I must admit that I've come to feel as much pride taking him to his dance studio as I would if we traveling to a Little League game.)

At first glance I find it sad that Aron is closeted, so to speak. At the same time, again, I stew over whether the inner tension I conveyed over the years has contributed to the situation. On the flip side there is something healthy about figuring out how to negotiate between expressing who you are (as though it were a static concept) and acclimating to the real world. We all learn to submerge certain aspects of ourselves depending on the context—didn't Freud write about that being a central component of the price we pay for civilization? During my former career in advertising I loathed the corporate world and what it stands for. Yet didn't I put these feelings away and develop the ability to slap a colleague's back and feign deep concern when sales of Ford F-150 trucks were off a point? I wanted to eat, after all.

On the other hand, what Aron is repressing is such a vital part of his very identity. Comparing the masking of my attitude toward big business as an adult with burying the conflicted sentiments my son has about gender as a child is almost to belittle what he must be going through. I can only hope that navigating this terrain is tolerable for him and that he isn't shouldering more than his share of pain.

He seems to get it though. On a recent visit with my mother, who lives four states away, she asked Aron why he was shielding his doll as he carried it.

"Well, Farmor" (Farmor is the Swedish name for grandmother, which she prefers to go by), he whispered. "A lot of people aren't open-minded!"

It sure took me long enough to get it. And when it arrived, it didn't suddenly appear in a flash of insight. No single event triggered it. The process was painstakingly gradual. Perhaps what ultimately helped bring me to acceptance was that slowly but surely, Aron started to exhibit more "boy" or at least gender-neutral behavior to go with his girl activity. He now enjoys save-the-world cartoons like *Ben 10* and *Generator Rex*. (Ironically, for a while I complained to Aron that he was watching too much violence, to which he would generally reply, "C'mon, you know it's just pretend"). He spends far more time building Lego kits and personally designed structures than combing the blond hair of his Hannah Montana doll.

Moreover, it's so much easier to talk with him about gender issues now that he's older and I don't have to scratch for the words that can reach a boy with a prekindergarten comprehension of the world. Of course, I no longer feel the need to broach the topic as often. A few months ago I thought I would check in with him.

"So, how do you feel about being a boy these days?" I casually inquired.

"It's okay, Papa," he nonchalantly assured me.

End of conversation.

Last year I finally felt ready to have what I perceived to be a necessary (albeit brief) heart-to-heart exchange with him. As I was putting my son to bed I began, "Remember how your mama and I have talked about people who aren't open-minded about boys who play with girls things—who just don't get it?"

"Yeah," he said.

"Well, I want you to know that I used to be one of those people—I didn't get it either. And I want to apologize for not being understanding and for the times I hurt you because I didn't accept you being different." I continued, "I love you Aron, and I love everything about you."

We embraced a good while longer than usual and then he crawled up into his bunk bed and went to sleep.

As a means of encouragement, I sometimes tell Aron how much fun it is to be different. I've always been so myself, not about gender but in terms of my ideological stance on life. At least since I was a teenager, I've been the perennial nonconformist, the person who—to paraphrase one of Groucho Marx's famous lines never wanted to join a group that would have me as a member. I have forever questioned mainstream assumptions and conventions. And I wouldn't have it any other way. On occasion, then, I share experiences with Aron about when I didn't go along with the people in the gang and didn't care what they thought about it—that maintaining my own convictions was more important. The point isn't to go against the grain for its own sake but to strive for a deeper veracity that no crowd could ever impart. The journey is inescapably personal.

Nevertheless, I wonder if I would have reached the point of acceptance had Aron continued with his persistent feminine expression—if he had insisted on dressing as a girl full-time or, harder still, had been adamant about becoming a girl. The guilt still rears its ugly head from time to time. And even now I have momentary setbacks when I find myself wincing at something Aron does or says.

Yet I'd like to think I would have come around. Surely I would have learned to set aside my discomfort and hypocrisy and celebrate my little wonder, right? Some essentials ring so much louder than others. The truth is, he is my son. He is my daughter. He is my teacher. He is Aron.

REFERENCE

1. Tuerk C, Menvielle E, de Jesus J. If you are concerned about your child's gender behaviors: a guide for parents [brochure]. Washington, DC: Children's National Medical Center; 2003. Available at: http://www.childrensnational.org/files/PDF/Departments andPrograms/Neuroscience/Psychiatry/GenderVariantOutreachProgram/GVParent Brochure.pdf. Accessed January 24, 2006.

Raising a Gender Non-Conforming Child

Deborah L. Wisnowski

KEYWORDS

- Gender non-conforming children • Support group

I was asked to write an article for this issue of the *Clinics* about my experience raising a gender nonconforming child and starting a support group for GNC children and their families. The timing of this request is interesting, because I've often sat down and tried to do just that but most times I quit after a page or two. I stop because I don't know where to start, what to share and what not to share, why I'm doing it, it's just too hard . . . or a million other reasons.

We all have challenges and until you walk in someone else's shoes, you can't know what their experience feels like. I've accepted what I'm affectionately calling "the challenge" to put my experience in words in hopes that my experience will help another parent with a gender non-conforming or transgender child, help an educator support such a child, and help a medical professional direct a family to the resources they may need. I'm writing from my perspective only and anything I say is my opinion and based on my experience and not those of any other parent of a gender non-conforming child. The decisions I've made and the paths I have taken were chosen based on my child's needs and were and are being made to make his/her life as productive and healthy as possible.

Sometimes it's hard to make sense of all that comes with raising a gender non-conforming child. I want to share with you with the confusions, frustrations, lack of support, love, and commitment to my child and other gender non-conforming children, as well as the changes I'd like to see in the medical and psychiatric community in treating these children. I believe we aren't given anything we can't handle and that all our challenges come wrapped in opportunity. Opportunity to change the way one sees the world, embraces life, and gives back, and ultimately the opportunity to make a difference in a life. My first priority is to make my child's life as good as it can be and provide the foundation he/she needs to live a successful life on his/her own.

Today, I am the mom of two teenagers, ages 17 and 15. My oldest is gender conforming and my youngest is gender non-conforming and always has been. In my journey to support my youngest, I am one of the founders of Stepping Stones, a

[a] Stepping Stones Support Group, NY, USA
[b] Parents, Families, and Friends of Lesbians and Gays, New York City Families of Color and Allies (PFLAG FCA NYC), NY, USA
E-mail address: debbywiz@yahoo.com

Child Adolesc Psychiatric Clin N Am 20 (2011) 757–766
doi:10.1016/j.chc.2011.08.003
1056-4993/11/$ – see front matter © 2011 Elsevier Inc. All rights reserved.

support group in New York City for gender non-conforming children and their parents, and I am on the board of directors of PFLAG NYC FCA (Parents, Families, and Friends of Lesbians and Gays, New York City Families of Color and Allies; www.pflag.org), who proudly sponsors our group. It's been quite a roller coaster ride and I'm anticipating it will continue this way for a while.

Looking back, it's hard to pinpoint when I really knew Bobbi (not her real name) was gender non-conforming, and it is only when I look back that I realize that some of his frustrations and anger may have had more to do with gender than they did with the actual situation at the time.

My first memory of anything unusual was Bobbi's attraction to headbands, nail polish, and his sister's toys. I have a Christmas picture of him at the age of two-and-a-half on his new Little Tike's race car bed, drinking a bottle, with a scattering of typical boy toys on the bed; but when you look more closely, you can see that he is holding a pink pocketbook.

Around the same time period, Bobbi began to wear headbands and a pair of penny loafers that he refused to take off. I wouldn't say the penny loafers were feminine and I never thought anything of his wearing a headband. He was just a silly kid. He loved Barbie and when I got my nails done, he wanted his done too and would be very upset if I wouldn't let him. A lot of the time I didn't let him. After all, boys don't wear nail polish, and his father was not too happy about it when I did let him. As Bobbi reached school age, he loved Barbie even more and that's all he wanted to play with. It was like an obsession. He had only one friend; a girl.

At this age, dressing became a problem, but he never asked for girls clothing and he hated most clothes. He would only wear jersey material pants and t-shirts. In the warmer months, he had a particular pair of red shorts that he loved. When he wore them he rolled them at the waist to make them shorter, and this was always a battle between us, because they were way too short for anyone and he looked bad in them. He would promise not to roll them but when I picked him up from school, they'd be rolled again. I wanted to throw them away but they were the only shorts he'd agree to wear, no matter how many stores we went to for new ones.

Although he never asked for girls clothing, many times I would pick him up from school and he'd have jewelry on or a big scarf wrapped around his neck. He'd claim his grandmother gave them to him and he had brought them to school in his backpack. I'm certain he meant to take them off before I picked him up, but most times he forgot. To this day, I still don't really know where all those accessories came from. He would fly into fits of rage if he had to wear khaki pants or a collared shirt.

During the early years of elementary school, there was a lot of rage, most times over almost nothing; in hindsight, however, there were bigger things going on inside Bobbi that I wasn't getting. It's sad to think about those days and how he must have felt. Those were difficult times for all of us. I was questioning what was really happening, but was so hoping this was a long phase and that one day I'd wake up and it would be gone. He couldn't tell me what was happening, either, because he didn't know himself or was afraid. I don't know why I didn't ask him more questions or why I didn't put this all together, but it wasn't long after this that it all started to come out. His interests remained unchanged throughout elementary school, but in fifth grade he really started to come out about who he is.

In fifth grade, Bobbi really started to work the accessories and started to reject male clothing and insist on girls clothes. He started to talk about himself more and say that he was a girl. He said when he was older he was going to cut off his penis. He begged to let his hair grow long. He had crushes on boys and was very open about it. He was happier then I'd ever seen him and Barbie finally disappeared.

There are many moments for parents of gender non-conforming kids that are heart-breaking and will forever be etched in our minds. Moments we pray so very much that our children forget. Moments we would change if we knew then what we know today. One of those moments for me was fifth grade graduation. The dress code for the ceremony was khaki pants and a collared shirt for boys—no exceptions. Bobbi was very upset about this, but I eventually was able to convince him to wear a pink collared shirt; I couldn't sell him on the khaki pants. He said, "I'm wearing my brown pants with the pink and silver stripe or I'm not going" and I agreed. The school would just have to deal with it.

We went to *Lord & Taylor* to buy him the shirt. On our way to the boys' department we had to pass through the girls' department, where Bobbi looked at the pretty dresses with envy and then turned to me in tears and said "I don't want to wear that shirt." By the time we got to the boys' dressing room to try on the pink shirt he was in tears and in a full rage. This was terrible: He was 11 years old and hysterical over a shirt—obviously there was more to this than I was grasping. He made it through graduation in his pink shirt and brown striped pants, but that shirt was ripped off two minutes after leaving the ceremony. Today, I wouldn't make him go and this year he graduates from middle school and he has already told me he will not be going to the ceremony. I didn't ask why; I know why. He won't be attending this time.

Graduation was supposed to be a time of celebration, of honoring a child reaching a milestone, looking into the future, a new school, new kids, and puberty. I should have spent that day proud of Bobbi, and I was. I was very proud of how brave he had become, how special he is and how much I love him, but more than all of those things I was scared and sad. I was really scared of all that lay ahead for him; even though I didn't really know what that looked like. I knew if this was his path it wasn't going to be easy. I was sad; sad that this was the burden he'd been given. It seemed so much for one little person. It seemed so unfair.

It was during the last half of fifth grade that I started to seek professional help for Bobbi and myself. Coincidentally at the same time Bobbi's school was assigned a new psychologist who took a liking and interest in Bobbi. Soon after spending some time with him, the psychologist contacted me and Bobbi's father—from whom by this point I was divorced—and asked us to join him for a conference about Bobbi. He recommended that we contact the Children's National Medical Center (CNMC) in Washington, DC, about the program they run for gender non-conforming kids. Some parents may have been insulted by such a conversation, but I didn't take it that way. I think he knew I needed direction and to find what support was out there. He also knew Bobbi's father wasn't supportive of Bobbi's gender non-conformity and may have felt this information may have been accepted more easily if coming from him instead of me. So I was grateful for his reaching out to me. He put me (Bobbi's father choose to not be involved at this point) in touch with the CNMC, which runs an online support group for parents of gender non-conforming children up to the age of 12 (see Dr. Menvielle's and Ms Tuerck's article in this issue).

The CNMC requires you go through a paid intake process to join. You are interviewed on the phone for an hour and a half by a psychiatric nurse. I made my call shortly after receiving the contact information and this call proved to be life changing for me. I was assured that there were many parents just like me and, along with a doctor and nurse, they were working together to help each other through the unique challenges we face through an online list-serve. After my acceptance into this group, I spent two days online reading past posts from parents about all the same experiences I was having. I laughed and I cried a lot, but I no longer felt alone. I now had people to communicate with who understood me.

So I had accepted that Bobbi was gender non-conforming and that I needed help navigating this journey. CNMC was a great resource, but I needed to work with a professional close to home to help me answer some of the questions I had. About the same time I contacted CNMC, I also contacted a child psychiatrist who specialized in working with gender non-conforming children. I am fortunate to live in the New York area, with access to some of the very few "experts" in this field. It's important to me that the professionals I work with are focused on this topic and have a lot of experience in this area. I had a lot of questions:

- What kind of support do I give my child?
- How do I keep him safe yet still allow him to be himself?
- What do you think is the outcome of this—will he be a transsexual?
- When do I have to look at next steps—puberty blockers?

It was important to me to have a professional guide this process wherever it was going to end up. He helps me to take all of this one day at a time and try not to look too far into the future, because we can't be certain what the future looks like. He is the voice of reason.

There are many challenges parents of gender non-conforming children and their children face. The hardest of these are social. With very few exceptions, our culture expects and is designed to support very binary gender roles. Being outside of those norms causes confusion and questioning by parents and children. Some of the challenges are:

- Who do you tell and why do you tell them?
- How do you tell them?
- How do you talk to people and get them on your side to support your efforts and protect your child?

It's not just that the questions themselves are hard to answer; the concern is what the outcome of this conversation is. And, once it's out there it can't be taken back.

I always thought about why would I tell someone first, and the answer to that was I needed them to support me and my child in the case of school administration, or I wanted them to support us in the case of friends and family. How to tell people is different for all parents—I am a very factual person and tend to share the facts first, instead of the emotional difficulties associated with my journey. I tell people what I know: That my child is gender non-conforming and has always been that way, which means he prefers female clothing, female play, and the company of girls. I speak to them from a place of confidence in myself, love for my child, support of who he is, and I probably, intentionally or not, leave no room in the conversation for them to question my decisions.

For those people who I need to help support my child, I ask straight up for their help and support. I tell them exactly what the challenge at the time is and ask them to help me. I generally know what I want from them, but I often let them make the suggestion first, because it is generally obvious what I'm looking for; but if they make the suggestion, it's their idea and that commits them to helping. If you tell the right people and create allies for your child, you will protect them. Always talk to those in a place to help you from a place of confidence in yourself and trust that they will want to help you. It's very important to surround yourself with supportive people who honor your child for who they are.

One of the biggest challenges is with parents in the community. My worst experience on this journey was getting a phone call one day from a close friend who'd just been speaking to a woman who was very social in the community. She called my friend specifically to discuss my child. She herself wasn't being cruel, but let my friend know that all the parents on the soccer field were up in arms about the boy in pink, and that what they were saying wasn't nice. To this day, this is still a challenge. Parents teach their children to be bullies: No child comes into the world hating another and no child is allowed to bully without family support. This speaks to the fundamental issue that we live in a world where gender norms are very binary.

As I write this, my child is now 15, on puberty blockers, and most likely on the path of transitioning to a female (see Dr. Wylie's article in this issue). Looking back, I can remember how big these questions were to me and how anxious I was even thinking about how to start some of these conversations, even with my family. Today, I don't really care what people think although I'm very careful about who I share my story with, not only socially but within the "professional" community, and I surround myself with people who are embracing of my child and my life. My journey is about my child and I believe anyone I share this with would do the same things I am doing; and if they didn't, they would be doing their child an injustice. You don't meet me on the soccer field or the PTA meeting, because this situation simply isn't that common.

All people face challenges in life, especially people with children. No one gets off that easy, and people can empathize with the family that has an autistic child, children with disabilities, or with medical conditions because they can be diagnosed: They are written about and accepted, with no one questioning whether they are real conditions or not, or whether the parent did something to cause this. But gender non-conformance doesn't have that medical validation. As a parent, I believe my child and all gender non-conforming or transgender children are born that way. However, I wouldn't have even thought about this topic if I didn't have a gender non-conforming child. Yes, it's all over the media today, but really I don't know any town where there is openly more than one child like mine.

The social challenges for a parent involve decisions for ourselves and our children, and as adults we are capable of making rational decisions and looking at our choices on multiple levels: How will this affect us today and tomorrow? Is this good in the long term? There are many questions. Unfortunately, the issues faced among our children are a little different, and for them, much harder—and can be overwhelmingly difficult for them to manage. Almost from day one, my child was gender non-conforming, and that behavior followed him to school where he was faced with many challenges, including his coming home stating "no one wants to play with me," "no one likes me," "I'm not like the other kids," and "no one understands me." These are heartbreaking moments for a parent. We want so much to make their world perfect and for others to just see them for the great kids they are, but we can't do that. Although my child always loved school socially, he is very misunderstood and isolated.

As Bobbi gets older, the tendency to isolate himself is getting stronger, and although he has friends in school, he never invites them over after school or spends any time outside of school with them. In elementary school, he had one friend and they were best buddies. They were both social "misfits" among the others and they found friendship with each other. This friendship lasted many years until, sadly, she became involved in drugs, which my child wasn't interested in. It was sad because my child depended on and needed her friendship. She embraced who Bobbi was without question and she is missed.

Trying to fit in and discover who you really are can take many of us down the wrong paths. These are lonely times for Bobbi and heartbreaking for me to watch, but I am proud that I raised a child who knows it's a safer decision all-around to sit home with me rather than trying to fit in with the "cool kids."

In addition to friendships, simple things like bathroom use became very uncomfortable as Bobbi got older and began to identify more as female. In elementary school, he went to school dressed fairly neutral and looked like a boy. Using the boys' bathroom was fine then. However, as he got to middle school he couldn't really maintain the neutral appearance, and there were new kids to contend with who didn't know whether he was a boy or a girl. He couldn't go in the boys' bathroom, because it's unsupervised and he could very easily be a victim of physical violence; and he certainly couldn't use the girl's bathroom. Even though at this point she presented very female, using the girl's bathroom wasn't a good choice for many reasons. How would the girls who knew Bobbi wasn't a biological girl react? How would the boys who knew he was a boy react? How would the parents react who heard there was a boy using the girls' bathroom? All of these questions made this an unsafe situation for Bobbi.

There are those within the groups of parents with gender non-conforming children who believe we should fight for our children to use the bathroom of the gender they identify with, but I am not one of them. I don't feel that this is a battle I'd want to fight, until and if my child transitions. I understand their reasoning of having their children as comfortable as possible, and that they know their children are the gender they are identifying as, so they should live as the people they really are. However, this is an area I wouldn't fight administration on because they have been so supportive along the way that I would not want to make it hard for them to support my child. If I begin to ask for things that create challenges for them internally and with other parents, then I might not get the little things that they do for us outside of what they were legally bound to provide. I don't want to risk that.

It's important to pick your battles, and today I just don't think this was one is important enough to fight. Even as Bobbi approaches high school, is on puberty blockers, and dresses as a girl, this is still not a battle I will take on. So, in an effort to keep my child safe, I made an agreement with the school to allow him to use the nurse's unisex bathroom or the unisex bathroom in the library. Bobbi is okay with this, and because of this arrangement, both the nurse and librarian are allies and protectors of Bobbi, which is invaluable.

Playing is hard. Boys are expected to play with trucks, get dirty, love video games, and love sports. Girls are expected to love dolls, dress up, playing mom, and be gentle. Although there is some accepted crossover, especially with girls, there is very little room for crossover with boys. Boys are looked at differently and negatively if they like dolls and not trucks, fashion and not sports. Girls are embraced for being a "tomboy." There is no "marygirl" in the world, is there? Why not? For as long as I can remember, Bobbi always played with girl toys and never ever picked up a truck. Without exaggeration, I'd spend hours at Toys"R"Us trying to convince him that action figures were just as cool and fun as that Barbie doll he always wanted. I would almost in desperation at times beg him to just listen to me tell him how interesting the toys in the boys' aisles were, and those in the artsy areas were, and that it was okay to like both boys' and girls' toys. But no. He wanted what he wanted and loved that Barbie.

Toy shopping was hard. I didn't care that he loved Barbie when he was just a child, and I would buy them for him. But at times he didn't want me watching him pick out a toy. He'd insist that I leave him alone to look around; of course I knew where he'd be and after a sufficient amount of toy shopping time I'd find him and tell him to make his final decision. He'd dance around his final choice; going back and forth between what I think he thought was a more masculine doll and the very feminine Barbie. I'd always tell him that he could get what he wanted and I was okay with either of them, but I could see his struggle.

I must have spent too much time trying to convince him there were other toys that were more interesting, and in doing so I sent him the message that "I wanted him to choose something else," or worse "This choice wasn't okay with me." Today, I'm sorry I made him feel that way. That was very unfair to him, but the truth is, I did want him to choose something else. I wanted him to walk in that store and pick an action figure, a video game, a ball, something blue, or even green—anything but Barbie. I wanted him to want a boys' toy. I did. I hated that doll. By the time she finally disappeared out of Bobbi's life, by his choice, I probably threw away more of them then I let him keep, hoping he wouldn't come home from school looking for her. Of course, there were so many of them that I could never get rid of all of them, and I wasn't always privy to the fact there was one traveling back and forth to school in his backpack with him. He loved her. Bobbi finally let go of her in fifth grade when he was allowed to dress in girls clothes at home and met other children like himself.

Playing at school is hard too. It was hard in elementary school because kids just automatically thought boys should play with one type of toy and girls the other. But with teacher intervention, kids got who Bobbi was and didn't care what he played with; and so for the most part elementary school was okay. Not great but okay. The school playtime gets harder once middle school starts. Physical Education programs are divided by boys and girls. If you are a gender non-conforming child, you may not feel you fit very neatly into that category, or worse you fit into the opposite category.

Middle school poses new challenges with physical education: The locker room! I had no problem getting help with this, but this was an area that if I had been told Bobbi had to participate in traditional physical education classes and use the locker room, I would have fought the school on. I would not allow my son in a locker room of preteen boys. This wasn't going to be a positive experience for Bobbi. Our school district likes Bobbi and has worked with us to make sure he was always protected. In fact, I had an "off-the-record" conversation with a school official who told me how I could keep him out of phys ed if an acceptable arrangement wasn't made for Bobbi. Bobbi was put into adaptive phys ed classes, which were taken at the same time as other phys ed classes but were "softer," with less aggressive sports, and did not require changing in the locker room. One of the arguments posed when discussing phys ed and bathroom use was that the school didn't want Bobbi to feel "different" from the other kids by not participating in phys ed and using a student's bathroom.

Middle school is a challenging time for all kids, as they try to figure out who they are among the pressures of being told who they should strive to be by their peers. They all want to fit in, be liked, and be popular. No one wants to feel different; but I challenge that I think gender non-conforming kids and transgender children do feel different, and let's face it, they are. Bobbi told me he knew he was different when he was two years old. So I'm not certain trying to have Bobbi fit in has any value.

One of the world's most popular "buzz words" is "acceptance." I interpret this as the idea that we should all believe we have a right to exist and live in peace with each other. I challenge the words "accept" and "acceptance"; I think they lack a commitment to learning what makes us different and therefore valuable. I'd like to see that changed to "embrace." Let's embrace the differences that we all have, and strive to learn from each other and respect each other. I like the concept and truth that "it takes a village to raise a child." The village takes care of everyone and no one in the village is left to fend for themselves. That's what we need in our schools: To learn about each other and support each other because of our differences.

As time went on, it became apparent to me that Bobbi's interests and behavior weren't changing. After joining the CNMC group and participating in a weekend get-together with families from across the country, I set out on a journey to start a support group in the metropolitan New York City area. I had met several families during that get-together who were interested in a group, and I took on the responsibility of trying to find us a place to meet. The child psychiatrist we work with offered us a room and was interested in helping us, but unfortunately the economy deteriorated, and his funding was cut, leaving me with nowhere to go. I reached out to another organization on Long Island who were also more than happy to help, but as our first meeting date approached, budget cuts were handed out and they too ended up with no funds to support keeping a room open for us to use.

After those two disappointments, which took over a year to set up and fail, I decided to reach out to the online group to try set up a meeting in the city with the kids. This worked okay and for a few months several of us from the metro area met once a month either at the zoo, a museum, or some other children's spot for a couple of hours. Although it was good to get the kids together and see the parents, it wasn't good enough. We needed a place to call our own, a room for the kids to hang out in and play and a place for the parents to sit and talk uninterrupted by the kids and other distractions.

During this time I met, under very "meant-to-be" circumstances, a woman who lived two towns away who also had a gender non-conforming child. It was wonderful to have someone to talk to who was so close and understood what I was going through. She got it! As a parent of a gender non-conforming child, it is hard to discuss what's going on with your child because no one gets it. It's hard to relate to if you've not experienced it and, as compassionate and loving as your confidants may be, they won't ever get it. Our friendship grew quickly, as did our kids' relationship. It was great for the kids to have each other: Someone to play with who didn't question why you liked the things you liked, and also liked them.

It's not always possible to expose your child to another gender non-conforming child, but parents should try to find this support. It helps children to accept themselves and understand that s/he isn't alone in the world, especially as s/he gets older or leans more toward being transgender. Such children are often the only child they know like themselves and are also very isolated. Imagine you're the only Jewish or African-American or Spanish child in your school or your work place. When you go home you are surrounded by other Jewish, African-American, or Spanish people: Your family. You have a place where you fit in. Now imagine you're a transgender child; when you come home you are still the only one like you. This can be a very lonely place for a child already overwhelmed by their circumstances.

As the friendship between parents grew, we were able focus on finding a place to hold a support group. After much searching, we finally met the woman who runs PFLAG NYC FCA who asked us to be on her board and offered us funding to pay for a room at the Center to start our group (the Center is the Lesbian, Gay, Bisexual & Transgender Community Center in Manhattan – ed.). She recognized the growing need for support of younger children and gender non-conforming children. It took a year and a half from my first phone call to get the group together, but it finally happened. Stepping Stones held its first meeting in January of 2010 and has grown from six families to over sixteen families. This is a private support group that requires a family to go through a free intake process to ensure that our group is an appropriate fit for their family. Most of our families hear about us from local professionals and are also part of an online support group.

We had many goals for the group, for both the kids and the adults. For the children's group, we had agreed that our children's lives were so much better now that they had each other that we wanted to provide this opportunity for other kids. Therefore, the children's group would be the focus of Stepping Stones. Stepping

Stones children's group provides an environment for gender non-conforming children ages four to fifteen to meet other gender non-conforming children, which very rarely happens within a child's home community. Many times, our children are isolated because of being misunderstood and don't have the opportunity to just play and be themselves. This is a safe place for gender non-conforming children to play with other kids without being questioned about their preferences of play, the clothes they are wearing, or the colors they like. We focus their activities on art, theatre, music, and creative play.

The children's group is a play group only, with no therapeutic component to it. However, it is run by a social worker with experience working with children and who has a commitment to the LGBT community. She donates her time to supporting our children, and plans the group's monthly activities. The families that we work with are very well-educated and supportive of their children, and if they feel their child needs therapeutic support, they take care of this need outside of the group.

In talking with other adults, it became clear that therapeutic support was not critical to a successful support group, but rather just being able to share experiences with other parents and to hear the different ways in which we all handled the challenges we faced on a daily basis was critical. Parents wanted to be able to talk about school challenges, social challenges with other kids and within their own families and friends, and share ideas with one another on how to handle the next steps. Based on the feedback we received from other parents and in talking to several professionals, we decided to self-mediate the adult group. We do invite professionals to join our group as guest speakers on occasion, which has been well received, but the group still agrees that we want to self- mediate.

We have also been contacted by many professionals and graduate students to come present to our group or to ask for our participation in their research studies. We welcome those who have a long-term commitment to the support and education of the world on gender non-conforming children to come present their projects to us; however, participation in the projects themselves is up to the individual families and is a private decision. As parents, our first role is to protect our children, and each family has to make their own decisions on how much exposure they are willing to allow into their lives. Research and education are crucial to changing our culture's perception of gender non-conforming children, and although there seems to be tremendous focus on this topic today, we are concerned as to the longevity of these efforts and those involved.

Our group continues to grow and change. I am looking to expand the group to include older children/teens, because Bobbi is the oldest of the kids and needs to meet older kids like himself. I am finding that it is hard to find kids and families his age. I know there are plenty of them out there and eventually this will all work out, too. That's the really great thing about our kids' group. Most of the kids are about the same age, so they will grow up together and always have each other. Bobbi is just a little more mature than the others at this point, so the search for different support is on again.

There are many frustrations in raising a gender non-conforming child. Many of them stem from the lack of resources and the fact that the resources available to us are so fragmented. The contacts I've made and support I've found have been on my own or through word of mouth. There is a very small body of "experts," but even among the experts there seems to be disagreement on how to proceed with treatment, especially as a child hits puberty. There seems to be no real authority and maybe there never will be because this is about human behavior.

With all the research and focus being given to gender non-conforming and transgender youth, I am hopeful that a more solid foundation is built on how to treat these youth medically and psychologically. I know my child was born this way, but I'd like to know *why?* Why is Bobbi transgender? What happened to cause this? I don't spend a lot of time on "why," but I would like to know. It might make life easier for Bobbi and his family. The world might embrace gender non-conformity if we could answer that question.

If I had one wish other than to take away this burden from Bobbi, it would be to spend one day as him. A person can share a lot about his or her life with you and you can think you know all about them, but you really don't. I know Bobbi has always had trouble putting his gender issues into words. I wish I could be him for a day so I would know all the right things to do for him and how it really feels to be him; when to hug him and cry for him and when to walk away and let him do it on his own. What does it feel like when he looks in the mirror? What does he see? Someone he likes and sees as having a good future ahead of him? What's it like to be in school—what does it feel like to know you are different from the other kids—or is this just how he is and he doesn't think about it? What's it like to not like your genitals? How's it feel to look at a girl and want to be one? What would I, as an adult, learn from this that could change his day-to-day life and his future?

When I'm with Bobbi I feel good. I'm comfortable that the decisions I'm making today for him are the right ones: That they will make his life better, that he will be able to focus on that life and not his gender, and that he will grow up to be physically and mentally healthy and that the steps I've taken medically will protect him emotionally and keep him safe until he's old enough to know who he really is and make the decisions necessary to live as he truly is.

As I write this, he's just started puberty blockers and although I struggled with this decision for a long time, it's the right one. My struggle really was about my hope that he would fit into the largest population of gender non-conforming children and just be gay, not transsexual, as he grew up. It seems like such an easier path. But he hasn't changed, and he isn't presenting or identifying as gay. In fact, several years ago during a car ride, Bobbi asked me, "When will I have to decide if I'm gay?" I told him he wouldn't have to decide, he'd know. That someday he'd want to kiss a boy or kiss a girl or that he'd fall in love with a boy or a girl. He said he thought he might be gay and we had a brief discussion about it. Several days later he came to me and said, "Mom, you know what we were talking about in the car the other day—well I don't think that's it—I feel like my insides don't match my outsides." I shouldn't have struggled so much. I should have just listened to him.

Considerations for Affirming Gender Nonconforming Boys and Their Families: New Approaches, New Challenges

Catherine Tuerk, MA, APRN[a,b,*]

KEYWORDS

- Gender identity • Children • Gender variance
- Pre-homosexual • Transgender • Homosexual

The media and the public's reaction have created the impression that gender variant behaviors of many children are indicative of later transsexual identities. This has suggested to some parents that the best way to manage their sons' gender variance, and perhaps gender dysphoria, is to allow them to dress as girls in increasingly more situations, to the extent that for some this becomes a transition to living full-time as a girl. This article poses some considerations in exploring these issues. Since I have had contact with relatively few parents of gender variant girls, I will not address these issues here. The issues of raising gender variant girls may be different from those if raising gender variant boys and require a separate discussion.

BACKGROUND OF THE GENDER VARIANCE SUPPORT GROUP: "FEELING GOOD, FITTING IN"

A support group developed through the Children's National Medical Center (CNMC) for parents with young children with gender variant behaviors started in 1998. The goal was to help parents help their children to "feel good" about themselves and "fit

---

This was written in 2007 when I was codirector of the program for families of children with gender variant behaviors at the Children's National Medical Center at Washington, DC. In January 2009, I resigned from the program at the Children's National Medical Center. I continue on as a consultant, conducting intake consultations for the listserv.

[a] Private Practice, Washington, DC, USA
[b] Gender and Sexuality Advocacy and Education Program, Children's National Medical Center, Washington, DC, USA
* 2605 Northampton Street, NW, Washington, DC 20015.
E-mail address: Catherinetuerk@gmail.com.

Child Adolesc Psychiatric Clin N Am 20 (2011) 767–777
doi:10.1016/j.chc.2011.07.005
1056-4993/11/$ – see front matter © 2011 Elsevier Inc. All rights reserved.

in" with social realities. We thought that a substantial majority of these boys would grow up and identify as gay, as all research has shown (cited elsewhere in this volume). Perhaps because of my own experience with my gay son, the many gay men whom I have known, and the research with which I was familiar, I had come to believe that the origins of sexual orientation were essentially biological. I was reacting to decades of mistaken beliefs that homosexuality resulted from the psychosocial environment (ie, too much mom, not enough dad). I did not believe that allowing a boy to express his feminine interests would cause him to later *become* gay but instead believed he was *born* gay. I thought that expression of feminine interests was part of the normal childhood development of many gay men. But I was also sensitive to the social environment of homophobia and heterosexism, and the prevalent belief that allowing a boy to openly express his femininity would stigmatize him. I hoped that our program would support or facilitate normal development with minimal shame.

A parent's guide (also developed at CNMC) reflected a positive, supportive approach to fully affirm and celebrate the child. This new approach was to avoid the necessity to correct and suppress the expression of femininity. The creation of many safe places for the full expression of gender variant behavior, primarily in the home, was encouraged. The initial group of parents in our support groups was resistant to allowing their boys to fully express their feminine interests, even at home. Parents were encouraged to develop a strategic approach for social interaction to minimize stigma. Dispelling the myth that there is or should be only one kind of boy became a central goal. Parents were encouraged to help the child understand the harsh realities of societal intolerance (ie, the macho standard of only one kind of boy). In 2003, we published the parent guide, based on the first 5 years of our experiences with the local parents' group.

Also, in 2003, Dr Edgardo Menvielle, codirector of the program, created a website and an email listserv at CNMC. At this time public awareness of transgender issues was increasing. We were aware of the work of the PFLAG (Parents, Families and Friends of Lesbians and Gays, www.pflag.org) Transgender Special Outreach Network (later the Transgender Network, or T-Net), and the Trans Family listserv, which were excellent resources for parents of transgender children (mainly adolescents and adults). Within our listserv, a few parents reported that their boys seemed to be excessively distressed and insisted that they were girls rather than boys. Many questions arose about how the childhoods of transsexual teens/adults may differ from the childhoods of gay teens/adults. Professionals began to question whether the diagnosis of GID (gender identity disorder) in childhood was appropriate to describe the common development of many gay boys, unnecessarily pathologizing children within the gender spectrum. It seemed there was a difference between the theatrical fun of gay boys playing dress-up and the stressful attempts of transsexual boys, who believed they were girls, presenting as their correct gender. One of my transsexual friends captured this difference when she said, "The gay boys want to be fabulous like Barbie; I just wanted to be like my mom."

In 2006, a trend began as more parents within the listserv felt their sons were transsexual girls rather than gay boys. This trend was initiated and supported by the intense interest in stories in the media of children beginning gender transition at early ages.

In general, there are 4 ways that parents deal with the challenges posed by their boys with gender nonconforming behaviors:

1. Forced conformity to masculine gender normative behaviors (the traditional oppressive approach).

2. Strategic compromise approach to dealing with social realities, as described in the parent's guide. In this approach, safe places, where feminine interests can be expressed, are established and distinguished from places where the child could be stigmatized.
3. The "free to be" approach allows children to dress and behave as they please, when and wherever they please. Parents choosing this approach are usually in more progressive situations where education about this issue is welcome.
4. The transgender or transsexual approach allows the child to pass as a girl or to begin a social gender transition from male to female.

We have helped many parents move beyond the first approach. Up to this time, the parents in the local support group have embraced the strategic compromise approach. We are confident that the first approach causes harm. We feel the second approach can enable most children to feel good about themselves and also face the social realities. We have little experience with the "free to be" approach and even less with gender transitions of young children.

GENDER DYSPHORIA AND VARIANCE IN MALES

There is considerable controversy around the issues of social categories of *gender identity* (as male or female), *variance* in associated gender behaviors (including sexual expression or orientation), and *dysphoria* (profound unhappiness) with the assigned gender. What do we think we know or believe that can help parents in raising their gender nonconforming children?

Historically and across cultures, societies have had a 2-gender system based on genitalia. A few societies make provisions for a relatively small number of individuals with another social gender role (ie, men acting feminine), and a few more allow individuals to live in a gender different from that assigned at birth (ie, men living as women). The specific content of the social gender roles varies greatly.

It is generally believed that more than 99% of the population is raised as either male or female and remains in that gender throughout their lifetime. The incidence of transsexuals, who began life assigned to one gender and at some time changed to live their life in the other gender, is currently estimated at about 1 in 15,000 to 25,000 and may be increasing. Biological males who are transsexual are predominantly conventional in their gender roles before and after their gender transition. However, there are also some transsexuals who are gender variant, either before and/or after their gender transition. The incidence of predominant homosexuality in males is probably about 5% (ie, 1 in 20). About two thirds of adult gay males report mild to intense gender variance in childhood, and an unknown but probably much smaller number report some history of gender dysphoria. Very few predominantly heterosexual males report a history of gender variance, although one fourth do describe themselves as being gentle boys.

When research began on boys exhibiting extremes of feminine behavior, most professionals anticipated that these males would later identify as transsexual. However, research studies have shown that a significant majority of these males actually identified as gay in adolescence or early adulthood. Various therapies had no effect on their later sexual orientation. However, the total sample size of these studies was relatively small and the men were still relatively young at the last follow-up. Based on the low incidence of transsexuality in the population, it is possible that transsexuals may not have been picked up in the sampling. In contrast, work with adult transsexual women has only found some, but not many, who would have been classified as "sissy boys" during childhood. Almost all transsexuals retrospectively report gender dysphoria during childhood, but few expressed themselves in a gender variant way that was evident to others.

The typical boy exhibiting extremes of feminine behavior shows a strong and persistent interest in the toys, play, and clothes of girls and a preference for girl playmates. He has an infatuation with hyperfemininity, including shoes, make-up, hairstyles, and anything feminine. He plays with Barbie dolls, not baby dolls, because this is not about nurturing a baby. He also has an avoidance of rough-and-tumble play. At a young age he may verbalize wishing to be a girl, or being a girl. The boy's gender variant behaviors seem to be playful expressions of creativity, fantasy, and beauty and are theatrical in nature. It is common for the expression of gender variant behavior to decrease later in childhood (around age 9 to 10), although it may again emerge during "coming out" in adolescence.

The typical gender dysphoric male, who identifies as transsexual in adulthood, reports that during childhood, she had an internalized feeling of discontent with being male (ie, dysphoria) and a desire to be female. She often did not engage in overt gender variant behavior. The initial coping strategy of these males is to try to be as conventionally masculine as possible. When this no longer works for them, they begin cross-dressing and seek to make a social transition by passing as females. Some of them may transition through the gay community, going through a period of time when they attempt to adapt by trying out being gay or presenting in drag (although their style may be more like a female impersonator than a drag queen). Some of them also go through a period of time in adolescence or adulthood (but not childhood) when they define themselves as heterosexual cross-dressers. The parents of most transsexual males also report that they noticed little that was feminine about their boys, at least before adolescence, and were shocked when their adult child disclosed a desire to change sex.

This information about typical patterns of gender nonconforming and gender dysphoric boys is based on experiences from the recent past, during a time when boys grew up in a highly stigmatized social environment of homophobia and transphobia. However, today we are in a cultural period of increasing acceptance of gay, bisexual, and transgender people, as well as a time of changes in the conceptualization of gender. So it is possible that these historical and cross-cultural incidences may change. Furthermore, positive, affirming parenting from an early age may have a huge impact. Whether the developmental patterns will change in this era of greater social acceptance cannot be determined until the present generation grows up. We do know, for example, that gay boys are coming out to others much earlier than in the past.

SOCIAL/SEXUAL BEHAVIORAL REHEARSAL

Two years is a common age when parents say they began to notice gender variant behaviors or feminine interests in their boys. At this age, children have idiosyncratic ideas of what it means to be a boy or a girl. Children learn about boys or girls from authority figures (parents and teachers) and from social cues, and they apply this knowledge to themselves. When they enter preschool and kindergarten, their notions of how boys and girls behave are concrete, highly conventional, and rigid. These gender classifications may generate questioning in a boy who is so different and even confusion about his gender identity. Although he knows he is a boy, he doesn't like the activities of other boys, and he does not see any other boys like himself—only girls. He does not realize that there are different kinds of boys, including boys who like girls' things. Also during childhood, children commonly rehearse social-sexual behavior that will fully develop later in adolescence and adulthood. A young gay boy may want to have a feminine presentation as a rehearsal for attracting the object of his affection (other boys). The fact remains that because of stigma we can only speculate about the normal development of a gay male. However, one could reasonably assume that if a person's love object is of the same gender and not the other gender, then that person's social-sexual developmental behavior would be different.

CONCERNS ABOUT CROSS-DRESSING AND SOCIAL TRANSITION

In affirmation and support of their sons with gender nonconforming behaviors, parents are often heavily influenced by the expressed desires of their children. Parents want their child to be happy and do not like setting painful limits. Parents want to affirm their child and to show they are not ashamed of him in public. For some parents and sons seeking to avoid the effects of the social stigma of gender variance, it seems to make sense to allow the boy to pass as a girl. Since young gender variant boys can usually pass easily as girls dressed in a skirt, this may be seen as a better (and/or easier) option than to be a boy with pink shoes and a Barbie doll in his arms. Other parents truly believe that their sons are "pretranssexual," and they wish to avoid the harm and pain that would ensue by limiting the child from living in the female role.

However, there may be possible pitfalls of allowing a boy to pass as a girl. We may contribute to gender confusion if it turns out that the child is not transsexual. We may limit the boy's opportunity to learn conventional male gender behavior. Boys who pass as girls may be forfeiting the opportunity to act on the realization that they can love someone of the same sex without changing their own sex. Some gender variant gay men have gone through a time when they thought they would be more successful in romantic and sexual relationships with men if they were female. This has been a motivation for some men who later regretted sex reassignment.

Unacknowledged homophobia-erotophobia may also relate to decisions to allow a boy to transition to live as a girl. In certain subcultures in the United States and Mexico, feminine gay men and transsexuals live together as females in houses for mutual support because of rejection from the larger culture, which does not tolerate feminine male homosexuality. In Muslim cultures, as well as more sexually liberal cultures like those of Thailand and India, it is much more socially acceptable for feminine gay men to live as women than to be seen as homosexuals. Religious pressure in countries like Iran results in gay men having sex reassignment surgery as an alternative to the severe penalties, including death, for homosexual behavior.

The World Professional Association for Transgender Health (WPATH; www.wpath.org) has guidelines for sex reassignment, which do not include cross-dressing in childhood. These Standards of Care include only living full-time as a female in adolescence and adulthood as a requirement for sex reassignment. Sex reassignment during adolescence is controversial but is gaining increasing support. Thus far there is no standard of care for gender reassignment in childhood.

TENTATIVE RECOMMENDATIONS

Liberal cross-dressing in general social situations and full-time living as a female represent totally new territory for boys with gender variant behavior. Because of this, a compromise approach may be the best first approach: Start by creating as many safe spaces for feminine expression as possible. Celebrate the child's interests. Give him lots of attention: it's no fun getting all dressed up without being seen and having interaction. Explain about different kinds of boys to normalize boys who like girl things, which will help him understand where he fits in the boy-girl scheme. Try to expose him to other boys like himself so that he knows that he is not the only one. Also expose him to adult male role models of different ways of being men. Be empathetic and supportive but set limits. In general, resist cross-dressing in public or passing as a girl.

If this approach does not work over a period of time, this may be indicative of significant gender dysphoria. If the child's distress increases and the "different kind of boy" concept provides no comfort or is consistently resisted and/or increases stress, then it is important to seek an evaluation by a professional with expertise in this area.

"DO YOU FEEL LIKE A BOY TODAY, OR DO YOU FEEL LIKE A GIRL?"

A parent new to our listserv reported this question as something she was advised to ask her son each day. She began to wonder about asking such questions. In this essay I will use the term "gender noncomforming" rather that "gender variant," which for many has become synonymous with transsexual.

I was giving a lecture to mental health professionals about gender nonconforming children and their families in Florida during November 2006. A mother came up and introduced herself after the lecture. She was the mother of "Jazz," a 5-year-old biological boy who had such profound gender dysphoria that his parents decided, with professional help, that he would transition socially as a girl. It had been 6 months since the story about Jazz had been published ("See Tom Be Jane," by Julia Reischel, in the *Village Voice*, May 30, 2006). A media blitz was in full force. We talked about Jazz. I had never heard a story like this before. I had never heard about such profound gender dysphoria happening at such a young age. We were both Jewish moms. She, like me, had tried everything. Her son's transition was probably life-saving. But she also shared my fear that perhaps too many people with gender nonconforming children would assume "transsexual" and would ignore the most likely outcome: "gay."

We had a lot in common, but her story was about success and mine was about failure. Her situation was immediately embraced by the transgender community; my situation was vastly different. On April 23, 1993, I had told our family's story in *The Washington Post*. There was also a media blitz at that time (I appeared on *Nightline* and *60 Minutes*, and my son was on *Larry King Live*), but it fizzled quickly. People were reluctant to face the fact that all human sexuality begins in childhood, and they certainly did not want to think about gay children. They much preferred the idea that some awful parenting style or sexual abuse were turning teenagers gay. Our story also stirred up anger and shame in gay men and their parents—no one wanted to talk about wanting to wear a princess dress and play with the ubiquitous Barbie doll, and they didn't want to hear our story of parents turning into "gender cops" and other forms of "physician-assisted child abuse." They didn't want to relive the pain. No one else, neither other parents nor gay people, were willing to talk about it. In contrast, the transgender community rallied around the positive story of Jazz.

Shortly after my son came out to us as gay, I tried to write a book about our story. I had an agent and several top publishers were interested. When my book proposal was sent around to some of the gay readers employed by the publishers to review gay-related ideas, the response was quick and extremely negative. One reviewer simply wrote the word "RETRO" in big red letters. Another said, "There is nothing that I find about this mother and her story that is admirable." It appeared that no one was ready for my story. It was too early.

PFLAG become my way to tell the story. Being president of PFLAG of the District of Columbia gave me an even bigger voice. Always in the back of my mind was the goal of starting a support program for parents of children like my son so that the abuse would stop. Like most people at that time, I knew almost nothing about transgender people—not until the question surfaced in PFLAG chapters all over the country, "Was PFLAG for GLB people or GLB and T people?" When the issue was introduced at a national PFLAG convention in the mid 1990s, I listened to the pros and cons. For me it was a no-brainer: of course our chapter was going to be transgender inclusive. I was totally shocked when I discovered that there were people on our PFLAG board who were very opposed. So we postponed the vote and engaged in a year-long educational program, which included professional speakers and people in the transgender community who shared their life stories. The stories were powerful. We all learned a great deal. I made transsexual friends, and our chapter had a transwoman who was our liaison to the transgender community and continues to be a close friend and adviser. I saw almost no connection between the childhoods of my transwomen (male to female) friends and my son's childhood. Not one person had reported playing with Barbie dolls and princess dresses. All were pretty conventional boys who harbored an awful feeling about their bodies and discomfort about their assigned gender. All had horrible childhoods and most didn't really become comfortable enough to transition until they were adults.

So when I was talking with Jazz's mother we both shared the dream that the horror could stop and it could stop in childhood—early childhood. After 5 years of being president of the transgender-inclusive District of Columbia PFLAG chapter, in 1998 I turned my attention to starting a support group for gender nonconforming children and their families. Thanks to child psychiatrist Edgardo Menvielle and the support of CNMC, our program became a great success. As the first program of its kind, it influenced the way people came to understand the childhoods of gender nonconforming children.

Over the past 20 years, I have probably talked with more than 400 parents about their gender nonconforming children; the majority of these were professional consultations with parents entering the CNMC's support group or listserv. During these consultations, I was always on the lookout for early gender dysphoria as described by transsexual friends and colleagues. I knew that some transsexual boys had a lot of feminine interests—not so much of the show-tune/Barbie doll/mermaid variety, but more the cooking/sewing/baby variety. Almost all the parents at that time focused on their fear of a gay outcome. I mostly looked for signs of dysphoria, boys feeling ashamed of and not liking their bodies, or opposite sex bathroom and underwear practices. Occasionally I would see a red flag. When I did, I would suggest to the parent to try the compromise/different-kind-of-boy approach. If that was met with a lot of resistance or increased anxiety, I would ask them to call me back and I would help them find a gender specialist to evaluate their child and provide professional guidance.

I also informed them of the only listserv that existed at the time, which was the Transfamily listserv created by Karen Gross, a PFLAG mother of a transsexual child. Later we created a special listserv for parents of girls. We also began a listserv for parents who may have had more gender-based concerns. We were able to find a core group of parents of gender nonconforming girls, but no core group emerged from the parents with significant gender concerns.

Although some of the parents in our local support group (which is small compared to the listserv group) had gender concerns, nothing surfaced that didn't seem to get resolved with age. As the children aged out of the group, the small number of parents with whom we stayed in contact reported that their children had identified as gay. Last year, parents of girls started coming to the support group for the first time. I understand that now the group has 1 child, aged 10, who is identifying as FTM transsexual.

By the time Julia Reischel's 2006 article appeared, the transgender community had come into its own. With the media blitz that followed her first article, *everything changed*. There seemed to be more parents who were willing to talk with the media about their gender nonconforming children. People in the transgender community were overjoyed (rightfully so) with the possibility that "pre-transsexual" children would be identified early and spared a childhood of horror. It was shocking for the public to realize that children were born in the wrong bodies, but in some way it may have been easier to deal with this "birth defect" phenomenon than the idea that gay children exist, perhaps because of the way people associate gay with sexual behavior rather than identity. After each major media presentation, requests to be on our listserv increased. Most parents were making the assumption that their children were transsexual. It became apparent early that there was conflation occurring between gay children and transsexual children.

It reminded me of what my longtime friend and mentor, Dr Greg Lehne, had told me about the early days of the Johns Hopkins Hospital gender clinic (the Sexual Behaviors Consultation Unit, started in 1971). When adult gender dysphoric people read about Christine Jorgensen's sex change operation in 1952, they finally understood what they had been feeling and the possibility that they could get help. But it wasn't just adults who were demanding care—it was also parents of gender nonconforming boys. Dr Richard Green decided that this was the perfect opportunity to study the childhoods of transgender people. He began his classic 15-year longitudinal study in the 1970s that ended, to his surprise, with the majority of gender-referred boys identifying not as transsexual but as gay, either at the end of the study or informally after the study ended. There was only 1 undocumented transsexual outcome.

This period since 2006, post Jazz, feels like a repeat of that history. Everywhere, lay people and professionals who tend not to know the history or have much experience in this area are making the same assumption—that gender nonconforming is equivalent to transsexual. The term "gender variance" has become synonymous with "transsexual" in many people's minds. I recently talked with Julia Reischel, who had been aware of the conflation that was happening. She wrote a second article, called "Queer in the Crib," that was published in the Pride Week issue of *The Village Voice* (June 19, 2007), 1 year after the first article. She was trying to remind the public not to overlook the little gay boys. It is interesting to note that the cover of that issue had a picture of a little boy dressed in leather with a whip, not a tutu.

After those articles, I decided to test the water by writing down my concerns and sending a early version of my *Considerations* paper, which precedes this essay, around to people I knew who were involved in this issue. Some were parents; others were activist friends and professionals (gay, straight, and transgender). The feedback was less than robust, which I interpreted as either they didn't agree with my concerns or they didn't like the informal format—not listing my sources—or they were afraid to upset the transgender community. Indeed, my transsexual friends informed me that in the transgender blogosphere, my concerns were being interpreted as transphobia.

I realized that the paper was a rather amateurish way of testing the water, but it did get people thinking. I am not an academic. I did not intend to write an academic paper, which is why I did not list my main sources. Most of what I have learned is from professionals in the field of gender and sexuality, my own experience as a therapist, and reading books, papers, and commentaries about people's lives. I have lived part of that life myself, being the mother of a gay son who was gender nonconforming in childhood. I am also re-living that experience through a child who is very close to me.

Three years have passed since I wrote the first version of the *Considerations* paper. I continue to have the same concerns. More and more parents are convinced that their gender nonconforming children are transsexual. More transgender listservs and programs are available. It might also be that parents are more aware of the red flags of gender distress. Maybe they are also more comfortable reporting and talking about the signs of dysphoria. Perhaps their children are more comfortable talking about these feelings with supportive and affirming parents. Perhaps something also is happening in the physical environment that is actually affecting our children. In the past few years, new research suggests that possible effects of environment chemicals may result in, among other things, an increase in male infertility and genital malformations in boys. Whatever the reasons may be, more and more children are being considered transsexual, and sometimes they are told about the possibility of being born in the wrong body during the "magic years," when fact and fantasy are very much commingled.

I fear that the normal stage of the development of gender constancy could be undermined or prolonged. By gender constancy, I mean the developmental milestone where the child realizes that his or her gender is generally fixed and does not change over time. This occurs somewhere between the ages of 2 and 7. Young children do not yet understand that people cannot change gender like they can change clothes, names, and their behaviors. Once a full understanding is attained, the child becomes increasingly motivated to observe, incorporate, and respect gender roles. This concept was developed by Lawrence Kohlberg, PhD. It has been and continues to be somewhat controversial. I am concerned that opportunities to help clarify the bewildering experience of gender nonconforming children may be missed or not reinforced enough. We know, for instance, that adopted children frequently fantasize that it was some imperfection in them that resulted in rejection by their birth mothers. We also know that children often fantasize that they were somehow responsible for their parents' divorce. We do not hesitate to clarify, consistently and repeatedly, their misconceptions in these situations. Although I appreciate the gender spectrum and the idea of gender fluidity, I feel it is easier for most children to be able to have some clear sense of gender, consistent with being either a boy or a girl. Like it or not, we depend on gender to make sense of our sexuality, society, and ourselves. I fear that prolonged gender distress will lead to increased high-risk behaviors during adolescence, such as seeking illicit hormones or silicone injections, drug and alcohol abuse, or suicide. I also know that no matter how much we try to help them clarify their gender issues, for some children it is simply not clear and not possible.

I do not want to sacrifice the life of one transsexual kid, but I do get concerned about the vast majority of gender nonconforming kids who are gay and not transsexual. I think we should always proceed with caution, knowing that for these kids, it is much easier to pass as a girl or be a girl rather than to be a boy who likes girl things. It would only be natural for kids who see no other kids like themselves, nor any adult role models, to be perplexed about where they fit in the world of boys and girls, and eventually men and women. They learn very early on that their way of being a boy is a problem for people, so they develop strategies to avoid the stigma and search for an understanding of themselves. This search is borne out by comments that children make:

"Maybe I'm half boy and half girl."
"Maybe I'm a girl on top and a boy on the bottom," or, my favorite.

"Maybe I just swallowed a girl" (which fits with the pregnancy fantasy of some young children).

Perhaps when we fail to clarify and explain how they might not quite understand and be perplexed by not seeing others like themselves, the issue remains muddled and disturbing. In my experience, many, but not all children, express relief when they can have a way of defining and understanding themselves as just a different kind of boy. Many gay people report remembering times of gender confusion when they were young. One lesbian patient reported, "I remember the exact moment, at around 8 years old, when I realized that I didn't have to be a boy to grow up and marry a girl." Many gay men also remember, as young boys, disliking their fathers' body hair and other masculine body features.

There is also new research and clinical observations indicating how mental disorders may impact or be impacted by intense gender nonconforming interests and behaviors. For example, concurrent conditions such as attention-deficit/hyperactivity disorder, bipolar disorder, anxiety disorders, and the autism spectrum disorders may make a child more vulnerable to social ostracism or gender confusion. This may help us understand some of the disturbing reactions that are so often reported by parents, such as emotional hypersensitivity, severe mood swings, oppositional behavior, temper tantrums, attention problems, anxiety, and depression.

I have also become more convinced after talking with parents that some of the intensity of the interests that we see in the boys is related to being talented in the arts, especially in graphic and theatre arts. This seems reasonable when we think about the huge contribution to the arts made by gay people. Most intense and persistent interests and talents seem to start early. I recently noticed an article in the July 2009 *Smithsonian* magazine in which an accomplished biologist, who specialized in the behavior of ants, remarked that his mother reported "that I looked at ants since I was in diapers." Imagine if his interest in science at an early age had been stigmatized!

In the past, many transsexual people, especially female-to-males, transitioned through the gay and lesbian community, identifying first as gay or lesbian, only to realize a transsexual identity. Today, with a greater visibility and appreciation of the transgender community, perhaps we are seeing an opposite trend. It seems as though gender nonconforming gay youth may be finding refuge in the transgender community, particularly in the minority communities where homosexuality is more stigmatized. Recently, the director of an inner-city transgender community program told me that in his group for transsexual teens, many were actually identifying as gay. This made him change the title of his group to be gay inclusive.

I remember a presentation at an American Psychiatric Association meeting about a social worker who worked with mostly black and Hispanic severely disadvantaged inner-city children. He had followed a couple of them informally as they resurfaced from time to time within the city's social service system. These gender nonconforming teens had found homes and affirmation in the transgender community. They had been highly homophobic and identified as transsexual. Many years later, the social worker had a chance encounter with 1 of the kids, now 26 years old. He had managed to overcome his tumultuous background, was gainfully employed, now identified as a gay man, and was living happily with a gay male partner.

I recently met a woman during a Pride parade. I was very excited to talk with her because she was the mother of a transsexual (MTF) teenager. She reported that when her now-daughter came out to her, she was absolutely unaware of any childhood gender nonconforming behavior or any gender distress, which reinforces the experiences of my transsexual friends who were also not interested in playing princess.

However, looking back, she thinks that perhaps there may have been some clues that she missed.

I am overjoyed that the lives of transsexual children have the possibility of being much better. An aware and affirming parent may pick up early clues and completely change the childhoods of transsexual people, so they do not need to develop the masculine or even hypermasculine defenses of denial and repression.

The WPATH Standards of Care guidelines provide a slow and thoughtful progression toward gender transition for adolescents and adults. With young children, it is hard to differentiate between impulsive survival instincts, inability to know how they fit into the world, and magical thinking without much ability to perceive what could lie ahead. Much research is now happening, including some started as part of our program at CNMC. Never before have we had the opportunity to study the outcomes of a large number of children (boys and girls) with gender nonconforming behaviors who have experienced positive parenting during early childhood. Things will become clearer. At some point we will probably be able to differentiate between transsexual kids, gay kids, straight kids, and some who will undoubtedly be somewhere in between.

In the *Considerations* paper, after consulting several sources, I wrote that the incidence of transsexalism was 1 in 15,000 to 20,000. Now, it is not uncommon for people to say 1 in 500. That is a big difference. If that incidence is referring to individuals across the gender spectrum with gender dysphoria, then perhaps it is reasonable. If it is meant to indicate the incidence of transsexuals, then it seems doubtful. Once again we are left awaiting more well-defined and agreed-on terms and more research.

It is remarkable and wonderful that the transgender community is finally receiving the recognition and acceptance that the gay and lesbian community enjoys today, even though it is still far from true equality. For years I have said that the painful stigma of being gay doesn't begin in middle school; it begins in nursery school. We can say the same for transgender people. But I am not sure that the gay "girly boys" are not once again being misunderstood, perhaps because of lingering homophobia, femphobia, erotophobia, and misogyny, just when the concept of "queer in the crib" was making considerable headway.

Recently, an article was published in *Scientific American* magazine entitled, "Is Your Child a Prehomosexual? Forecasting Adult Sexual Orientation" (September 15, 2010). Could this be a sign of the "comeback kid?"

Improving Medical Education About Gender-Variant Youth and Transgender Adolescents

Joel Stoddard, MD, MAS[a,b],*, Scott F. Leibowitz, MD[c],
Hendry Ton, MD, MS[a], Shane Snowdon[d]

KEYWORDS

- Gender identity • Gender nonconformity • Gender disorders
- Medical education • Continuing medical education

Gender-variant youth (children and adolescents) and transgender adolescents have in common expression and/or experience of gender that does not conform to societal expectations. For brevity, we refer to them as gender minority youth, although they are not identical in phenomenology or outcome. See the article by Pleak elsewhere in this issue for further exploration of this topic. In addition, although often lumped together with sexual minority youth as the T of LGBT (lesbian, gay, bisexual, transgender), gender minority youth present at different times with unique problems (**Fig. 1**). Stigma related to gender nonconformity may drive adverse outcomes in these youth,[1,2] and, like sexual minorities, transgender adults receive less family support.[3] Thus, a general guideline for clinicians who work with gender minority youth is to reduce these youth's overall experience of stigmatization, promote their resilience to stigmatization, and facilitate family adjustment.[4]

Since the American Association of Medical Colleges (AAMC) issued a policy statement promoting education for competent care for LGBT individuals in 2007,[5] there has been an effort by the AAMC and others to assess the prevalence and quality of LGBT education across the country. Notably, the Stanford School of Medicine

The authors have nothing to disclose.
[a] Department of Psychiatry and Behavioral Sciences, University of California, Davis, Health System, 2230 Stockton Boulevard, Sacramento, CA 95818, USA
[b] Section on Bipolar Spectrum Disorders, Emotion and Development Branch, National Institute of Mental Health, Building 10, B1D43B2, Bethesda, MD 20892-2670, USA
[c] Department of Psychiatry, Children's Hospital Boston, Harvard Medical School, 300 Longwood Avenue, Boston, MA 02115, USA
[d] Center for LGBT Health and Equity, University of California, San Francisco, USA
* Corresponding author. Department of Psychiatry and Behavioral Sciences, University of California, Davis, Health System, 2230 Stockton Boulevard, Sacramento, CA 95818.
E-mail address: leoj@alum.mit.edu

Child Adolesc Psychiatric Clin N Am 20 (2011) 779–791
doi:10.1016/j.chc.2011.07.008
1056-4993/11/$ – see front matter Published by Elsevier Inc.

childpsych.theclinics.com

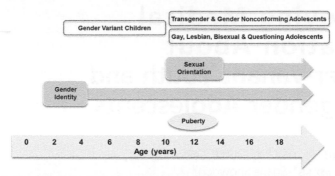

Fig. 1. Gender identity and sexual orientation development, presenting populations (light-colored boxes), and developmental tasks (gray boxes) are arranged along a timeline. Of note, sexual orientation develops later than gender identity, resulting in different ages of presentation. Gender variance has a wide clinical presentation in childhood, and what it predicts for an individual is unknown. Identities become more resolved during adolescence, where they are broadly grouped here according to gender identity and sexual orientation.

LGBT Medical Education Research Group surveyed all United States and Canadian allopathic and osteopathic medical schools. At the 2010 AAMC annual meeting, they reported that a majority (70%) of respondents assessed their LGBT curriculum as fair, poor, or very poor. No such comprehensive assessment exists in postgraduate medical education. There, gender identity issues may be addressed as a specialty area, for example as part of gender development issues in psychiatry or as part of sex hormone regulation in endocrinology. Some surveys of postgraduate medical trainees demonstrate that they are unaware of key needs of LGBT patients and are uncomfortable delivering care.[6–8]

When developing specific content and treatment recommendations, educators are challenged by current dilemmas about conceptualizations of pathology in gender minorities[9] and lack of evidence-based treatments for children who may meet criteria for gender identity disorder (GID) in the *Diagnostic and Statistical Manual of Mental Disorders* (DSM-IV).[10] Moreover, educators may be stymied by the paucity of research about gender minority youth relative to those who are sexual minorities. Even so, there are substantial educational opportunities for medical clinicians at all levels as well as established practice guidelines and educational resources. In this article, we describe our efforts to educate medical professionals at all levels about gender minority youth, offering suggestions to facilitate this process. We begin by describing a basic needs assessment and discussing promising, currently available educational resources to help educators get started. Next, we describe special issues and approaches to education for three levels: medical school, postgraduate training, and continuing education for practitioners. Although detailing specific recommendations is beyond the scope of this article, we suggest some specific teaching points and methods as well as institutional environment changes to help educators get started.

NEEDS ASSESSMENT

The general description of needs is usually required for grants, curricular changes, or other initiatives. In general, current research suggests that the psychosexual outcome of gender-nonconforming children, especially when meeting DSM-IV criteria for GID of childhood, cannot be predicted.[11] However, outcome data are clear for transgender adolescents. Evidence supports that they are at risk of psychosocial stressors and negative psychosocial adjustment; especially concerning are associations with high rates of suicide, survival sex work (prostitution), and human immunodeficiency virus infection.[2,12–20] Compared with sexual orientation minorities, transgender adults report less access to health care and more experiences of prejudice with physicians such as blaming, harsh language, rough treatment, and the use of excessive precautions.[21,22] Health care professionals are not necessarily prepared to work with these populations. From a policy standpoint, several prominent organizations have acknowledged disparities in health care for LGBT patients. These organizations include the AAMC, American Medical Association, Institute of Medicine, the Joint Commission, and the US Department of Health and Human Services. For medical schools, the University of California, San Francisco (UCSF) Center for LGBT Health and Equity offers a tool for institutional self-assessment vis-a-vis LGBT issues.[23] LGBT youth themselves have indicated more concern about receiving knowledgeable care (eg, demonstrating competency, a nonjudgmental stance, and listening skills) than about their providers' sexual orientation or gender identity.[24]

RESOURCES

Several practice guidelines exist or are in development that educators may refer to when learning about the field and deciding how to develop identified competencies. The oldest and best articulated practice guidelines are issued by the World Professional Association for Transgender Health (WPATH), which addresses children and adolescents with regard to distressing/impairing gender nonconformity and cross-gender identification. These guidelines are known as the Harry Benjamin International Gender Dysphoria Association (HBIGDA) Standards of Care, now in its sixth edition.[4] In addition, the Endocrine Society has developed clinical guidelines for transgender hormone therapy.[25] Practice parameters are in development for the American Academy of Child and Adolescent Psychiatry, which will more explicitly expand the approach by mental health professionals. These parameters are discussed elsewhere in this issue by Adelson. A summary of the available practice guidelines relevant to gender minority youth appears in **Table 1**.

Other than practice guidelines, there are several other resources for medical educators and practitioners. For practitioners interested in managing gender minority youths' gender issues, education may be needed that is even more specific (eg, specific hormonal treatments and psychotherapeutic modalities). For these practitioners, regional practice guides, practicums, and specialty clinic protocols are available. Medical educators and others may be more interested in basic competencies relating more to assessment and referral. Rather than being a special topic, this more general education about gender minority youth will likely occur in the broader context of LGBT education. To that end, modules have already been created for medical education at all levels about LGBT individuals relevant to gender minority youth. (See **Table 1** for a list of these resources.) In addition to these resources, later we suggest how this material may be integrated into existing curricula and taught.

TEACHING ABOUT GENDER MINORITY YOUTH IN MEDICAL SCHOOLS

Medical schools are ideal for preparing clinicians for a proper approach to gender minority youth. Although the topic may be approached as a standalone special topic, we prefer integration into the existing curriculum (see **Table 1** for content resources) and for the most part, key points and competencies have been identified. After

Table 1
Content and training resources regarding transgender and gender-variant youth

	Organization	Available at (URL)
Practice Guidelines	World Professional Association for Transgender Health: Harry Benjamin International Gender Dysphoria Association Standards of Care	http://www.wpath.org
	The Endocrine Society	http://www.endo-society.org
Specialty Clinic Protocols	Children's National Medical Center: Gender/Sexuality Development Program[a]	http://www.childrensnational.org
	Callen-Lorde Community Health Center	http://www.callen-lorde.org
	Tom Wadell Health Center	http://www.sfdph.org/dph
	Vancouver Coastal Health Transgender Health Program	http://transhealth.vch.ca/
Online Training Modules	The Fenway Institute	http://www.fenwayhealth.org
	The Association of Gay and Lesbian Psychiatrists and the Group for the Advancement of Psychiatry LGBT Issues Committee: LGBT Mental Health Syllabus	http://www.aglp.org/gap/
Texts/Publications	de Vries A, Cohen-Kettenis P, Delemarre-van der Waal H. Clinical management of gender dysphoria in adolescents. International Journal of Transgenderism 2006;9(3):83-94.	
	Ettner R, Monstrey S, Eyler A, editors. Principles of transgender medicine and surgery. Binghamton (NY): Haworth; 2007.	
	Makadon HJ, Mayer KH, Potter J, et al, editors. The Fenway guide to lesbian, gay, bisexual, and transgender health. Philadelphia (PA): American College of Physicians; 2008.	

[a] The Children's National Medical Center Gender/Sexuality Development Program has an outreach arm, the Gender and Sexuality Advocacy and Education Program, which maintains a list of resources and online groups for families.

mapping the curriculum, educators will find that this material may easily be integrated into existing topics. Several key areas for revision include infectious disease, mental health, sexuality, endocrinology, cultural competence, patient panels, health care policy, and professionalism. By way of example, the UCSF LGBT Center for Health and Equity has published a list of the LGBT curriculum infusions at the UCSF School of Medicine (found at lgbt.ucsf.edu). This type of comprehensive approach prepares students to competently consider gender minorities as a matter of course, because they will eventually be expected to do in practice.

We recommend using a cultural competence training approach to medical education about gender minority youth because the concept has already been formulated to address practitioner bias, gender, diversity, and differing belief systems.[26] One of the authors (H.T.) collaborated with medical educators, LGBT advocates, and trainees at University of California, Davis, to integrate the AAMC's Tool for Assessing Cultural Competence Training (TACCT)[26] adapted for LGBT training across all 4 years of medical student education in a planning retreat. The retreat sought to accomplish several goals critical to implementing LGBT curriculum:

- Organize key stakeholders into a single forum to maximize collaboration.
- Present and discuss a compelling rationale for an LGBT curriculum to establish "buy-in."
- Review the current cultural competence curriculum to ensure optimal integration and synergy.
- Review the LGBT learning content currently in the curriculum and LGBT learning content offered through outside resources (ie, online, textbooks, experts) in order to be familiar with starting resources.

The stakeholders then worked in small groups to map the TACCT competencies through the 4 years of training and to suggest methods of teaching and assessments. Thus, we have been able to integrate a plan for including education about gender minority youth in medical education considering the students' experience. A report of this integration is in preparation and may serve as another model.

Faculty who teach these topics may not have knowledge, experience, or comfort with gender minority issues. Knowledge is easiest to address and should not be overwhelming, because many have distilled key teaching points. Some may not be comfortable with gender minority issues or practiced with modeling a gender-neutral approach. The cultural competency education model addresses this by encouraging an open stance as well as awareness of bias and fallibility. Cultural competence educators who are comfortable discussing race/ethnic minority issues may, however, maintain unconscious biases toward gender minorities. These educators may have a high level of motivation to address these biases if given the appropriate forum for discussion and education. Faculty may draw on their experiences of learning to care for different patient populations. Similarly, faculty need to be aware of their biases and how they relate to challenging gender minority competencies before they approach medical students. As such, faculty may want an opportunity to discuss among themselves their comfort about material that challenges gender role assumptions. Gender role assumptions develop early, are usually entrenched, and are culturally transmitted.[27] This practice may be helpful before leading discussions with medical students, who may be more inexperienced at challenging their own assumptions.

TEACHING RESIDENTS ABOUT GENDER MINORITY YOUTH

As opposed to medical school, trainees in residency programs both practice medicine and are preparing for a specialized practice. In addition to the competencies that are required for medical students, they will need more detailed clinical knowledge and skills. As they are in practice, they will also need to be familiar with their local health care system.

Curriculum development for each type of residency is beyond the scope of this article. (See **Table 1** for a list of prepared specialty-related teaching modules and curriculum models.) In addition, some specialty clinics that serve gender minority youth offer externships to residents and medical students. Elsewhere in this issue, one of the authors (S.L.) describes the creation of a specialty clinic.

Residents, faculty, and practitioners need to be aware of systems issues as gender minority youth present for care. All practice guidelines recommend that prepubertal gender-nonconforming children who are impaired or distressed by gender nonconformity be assessed by a mental health practitioner trained in child development. Thus, it is important to identify mental health practitioners in the community who are able to assess a child and either provide care or make appropriate referrals. Residents should be aware that transgender adolescents will likely be treated by a group of providers including a general medical practitioner (pediatrician, internist, endocrinologist), a mental health professional, and possibly a surgeon. If identified as one of these providers, the resident and supervisor should be aware of the WPATH HBIGDA Standards of Care and their responsibilities to the patient.

Residents and practitioners should be aware that gender minority youth face stigmatization from several sources, and both the youngster and the family require support. They need to assess for bullying and may need to support school interventions. (See **Table 1** for several resources for gender minority youth and their families.)

CONTINUING MEDICAL EDUCATION ON GENDER MINORITY YOUTH

Practitioners who take advantage of continuing medical education (CME) activities are generally a self-motivated, active audience seeking to improve clinical skills. Generally, these practitioners are interested in achieving the competencies suggested for medical students, as well as the systems and practice issues described for residents.

Providing a formal CME course involves becoming certified by the state medical board to dispense continuing education units to participants. This step is often opaque to course coordinators operating under the auspices of a professional meeting or through a professional journal because this is done by the organization's staff. Many medical schools are affiliated with administrators who may guide individuals through the process and help inexperienced coordinators create education events such as symposia. To assess demand, promote their course, and aid in drafting a needs assessment, coordinators should consider affiliating with local LGBT advocacy groups. Content experts may be recruited from specialty clinics (see **Table 1**) and networking groups (**Table 2**).

However, CME need not be formal. Self-motivated regional practitioners treating gender minority youth become content experts themselves, often educating peers during luncheons and local meetings. This informal education promotes both access for gender minority youth and the provision of a referral base. Such practitioners have a variety of resources available to them from clinical protocols (see **Table 1**) to networking opportunities (see **Table 2**).

Table 2	
Networking opportunities for professional development for gender minority youth	
Medical Education	Gay and Lesbian Medical Association: Transgender Healthcare Committee
	American Medical Student Association: Gender and Sexuality Committee
	University of California, San Francisco: Center for LGBT Health and Equity
	American Academy of Child and Adolescent Psychiatry: Sexual Orientation and Gender Identity Issues Committee
	Lesbian and Gay Child and Adolescent Psychiatric Association
Clinical Care	World Professional Association for Transgender Health
	American Academy of Child and Adolescent Psychiatry: Sexual Orientation and Gender Identity Issues Committee
	American Association of Pediatrics: Committee on Sexual Orientation and Adolescents
	Association of Gay and Lesbian Psychiatrists
	Gay and Lesbian Medical Association

THE EDUCATIONAL AND PRACTICE ENVIRONMENT

The 2007 AAMC policy statement[5] on LGBT needs recommends that medical schools adopt nondiscrimination policies protecting gender minority individuals, develop curriculum promoting LGBT competence, and provide support for LGBT role models. However, the medical facilities in which providers and medical students work are unlikely either to have a nondiscrimination policy for gender minorities or provide LGBT competency training.[28] These institutions can promote equitable, inclusive care for LGBT patients in a variety of ways. A good starting point is a nondiscrimination statement that includes "gender identity and expression" as well as "sexual orientation," that is posted for maximum visibility to patients and employees and that is backed by clear complaint procedures. To promote compliance, LGBT competency training should also be available for all sites and staff. Institutions can also allow LGBT patients to identify as such in admitting, registration, and medical interviews, permitting gender minority patients to indicate their preferred name and pronoun if these differ from their medical record. Institutions can also consider adding transgender coverage (ie, for sex reassignment) to their employee insurance plans, because the great majority of plans now exclude transsexual care. Office and waiting area decorations should not be overlooked: for example, safe space posters, available from groups such as the Gay, Lesbian, and Straight Education Network (www.glsen.org) and Parents, Families and Friends of Lesbians and Gays (www.pflag.org), explicitly invite youth to discuss gender identity issues, among other subjects.

With regard to medical school and postgraduate training, a plan for mentorship and faculty development should be implemented. Currently, there are few transgender medical educators. More broadly, LGBT faculty and students may well be underrepresented in medical education at all levels. Therefore, medical students, residents, and faculty have few opportunities to challenge LGBT and gender bias among peers. LGBT students without role models may be repeatedly challenged by the anxiety of disclosing their sexual orientation or gender identity in various settings. Without proper role models for professional comportment, they may struggle in maladaptive ways. In addition to harming professionals who are sexual and gender minorities, a professional culture of heterosexism, sexual stigma, and gender stigma will adversely affect patient care.

There are several opportunities for mentorship and faculty development. Here faculty development and mentorship for LGBT-identified individuals are discussed. Issues related to readying faculty to teach about gender minority youth are also discussed. LGBT faculty, students, and allies who are identified should be encouraged to form a community connected by an e-mail list or social media and to meet regularly or at special outreach events. Targeted programs within the institution may address issues of disclosure of sexual orientation and gender identity, legal and financial challenges, career obstacles, and immigration concerns. LGBT faculty and students may be explicitly included in orientation programs, student life panels, professional development discussions, and social activities. Faculty and students should be made aware of mentorship opportunities through support organizations and meetings (see **Table 2**).

APPROACHES TO TEACHING

Educating clinicians in hospital and clinical settings on issues pertaining to gender identity and nonconformity can be broadly classified into didactic instruction and clinical supervision. This section explores modalities and suggests objectives. We provide suggestions on how to structure didactics and supervision. These suggestions are not meant to supplant more detailed descriptions of assessment and treatment described elsewhere in this issue.

Any didactic instruction on typical child and adolescent development should include gender and sexual identity development. Incorporating both the typical and atypical biopsychosocial pathways of gender and sexual development provides a framework to understand gender and sexual minorities as nonpathologic variants of human development (see **Fig. 1**). We also suggest a tool (**Fig. 2**) by which a trainee may organize the source of distress of a gender minority youth who may present for clinical treatment by visualizing those factors along a spectrum that spans invalidation and acceptance. Together these visual aids help organize a trainee's consideration of internal and external factors leading to the clinical presentation of a gender minority youth along a developmental continuum. In the case studies that follow, we provide two examples of how these tools may be used.

Subsequent didactic instruction on the development of psychopathology in gender minority youth should emphasize that gender minority status is not a pathologic state. Trainees should be made aware of unique issues faced by this population, the risks and protective factors, and the increased rates of comorbidities. For example, the presence of a physical-mind gender discordance in addition to family rejection suggests a specific clinical issue (internalized gender prejudice) coupled with a risk factor (family rejection), which may lead to the development of depression. In this example, internalized stigma, family rejection, and depression may each be a point of intervention. Comorbid psychopathologic conditions (eg, depression, substance abuse, suicide attempts) may arise as a result of risk factors related to gender minority status. These conditions should be distinguished from others (eg, pervasive developmental disorders, obsessive compulsive disorder) that complicate the diagnostic questions. Understanding and discussing the difference between the two should take place when teaching about psychopathology and gender minority youth.

Training programs routinely incorporate case conferences into their educational curricula. Inclusion of at least one case on gender variance (distinct from sexual

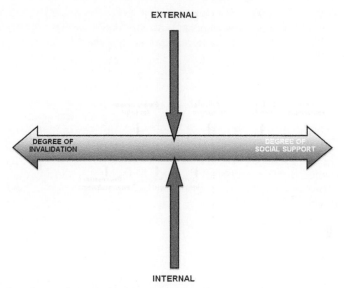

Fig. 2. Template for sorting gender identity issues along two dimensions.

orientation status) would expose trainees to the practical issues faced by clinicians when treating gender minority youth. There are several important points of discussion here. First, for prepubescent children, gender identity is fluid, and its impact on families remains crucial to the clinical approach when a patient presents for treatment. Second, there is no evidence-based approach to predict the adolescent outcome of a gender-variant child. This remains the hallmark dilemma in the treatment of these children. Finally, for transgender adolescents treated with puberty-blocking agents or cross-sex hormones, there are established phases of treatment (both medical and psychiatric) according to the Endocrine Society guidelines[25] and the WPATH HBIGDA Standards of Care.[4] At the end of this article, the authors provide several sample case vignettes for discussion. In addition to case vignettes, films have been frequently used to illustrate material (for examples, see the Web site of the Lesbian and Gay Child and Adolescent Psychiatric Association: www.lagcapa.org).

A training program or institution may also enhance "gender competence" through a single presentation, workshop, or symposium or integration into an existing seminar series. This approach may alleviate the need for an in-house staff considered competent or an expert in the field of gender identity. A benefit of large presentations is broad exposure to a larger audience. The limitation of relying on a single presentation as an exclusive or one-time educational event is the inherent time restriction, forcing more superficial coverage of the material. Educational materials about gender minority youth may be integrated into existing regular seminars in addition to those about human sexuality and gender development. Candidate seminars can include family and group therapy, psychosomatic psychiatry, and inpatient psychiatry settings. All presentations should provide attendees with access to resources following their completion (see **Table 1**).

Whereas didactic instruction lays the groundwork for the knowledge of the clinical issues in treatment, their application requires the responsibility of treating a gender

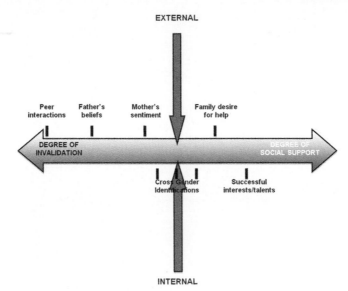

Fig. 3. Formulation of Case 1.

minority patient. The following two cases illustrate how a provider might apply this knowledge in the assessment and treatment of gender minority youth.

CASE VIGNETTE 1: A GENDER-VARIANT CHILD

A family with a 6-year-old boy named Brian presents to a clinician because Brian has strong "feminine" interests. "Our boy does 'girl things,' and we don't know what to do," his mother explains. These interests include playing with dolls and drawing female characters, some of which he makes up. He has expressed a wish to be a girl, especially when he was in kindergarten. The parents disagree on how much these behaviors are present. The father says that he does not see it that much. However, he recognizes that he has not been able to engage Brian in "guy activities" like tossing a ball or watching sports on TV. The mother is much more likely to witness these behaviors. Brian has an older brother, aged 10, who is "all boy." The mother says that Brian has been teased in school, and the teacher has told him he is not allowed to play with "girl things." Both parents seem uncomfortable and confused, and they want you to tell them what to do.

Brian's provider may approach the case by parsing the various degrees of invalidation and acceptance (**Fig. 3**). In addition, several clinical points are illustrated by this case. Brian's provider should recognize that it is very likely that Brian's mother and father have different approaches to him. This will help direct the provider to having separate discussions with them regarding their individual struggles about having a child not live up to their respective expectations. Brian's provider should also be aware that Brian may be suppressing his cross-gender identifications by differentially conforming to different peoples' expectations. For example, his father may "not see it that much" because Brian may be sensitive to his father's rejection and therefore suppress his cross-gender behaviors and statements in front of his father, which is typical of a 6-year old gender-nonconforming child. Brian himself likely feels ambivalent about his nonconforming gender identifications. In some instances those

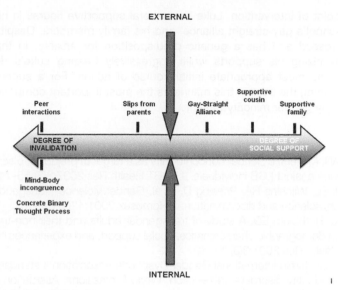

Fig. 4. Formulation of Case 2.

behaviors are comforting, whereas in other instances Brian suffers the ramifications of bullying and victimization. A treatment plan that addresses all the external and internal factors along the spectrum of invalidation and support should prioritize those interventions according to the severity and causes.

CASE VIGNETTE 2: A TRANSGENDER ADOLESCENT

Luke (born Lisa), a 16-year-old white biologic (natal) female, is now an affirming male who presents at the request of an endocrinologist. The endocrinologist needs psychiatric clearance initiation of cross-hormone treatment. "I want you to approve the testosterone treatment," Luke demands. Luke has had chronic depressive symptoms throughout his life. He reports identifying more as a male ever since kindergarten, although at the time he was unaware that he could do anything about it. In the eighth grade he went to Gay-Straight Alliance meetings at his school after coming out as gay. However, he realized soon after that he was actually transgender and not gay. He then told a supportive female cousin, but telling his parents was very difficult. Ultimately, he started seeing a gender therapist and began taking on the male gender role with support from his family. His father sometimes slips and calls him Lisa. There is a strong family history of anxiety. Despite reporting worthlessness, helplessness, hopelessness, passive suicidal ideations, and poor concentration, Luke was very up-front at the intake evaluation: "I don't need those stupid happy pills. All I want is my testosterone and surgery!" Despite living in a supportive home environment as a male, he continues to have poor sleep and is irritable. The parents report that he is unable to enjoy activities and focuses only on his transition.

As in the previous case, Luke's provider may begin by understanding the various degrees of invalidation and acceptance to identify points of intervention (**Fig. 4**). Luke's focus on hormone intervention is understandable, given the persistent lifelong discordance between his gender identity and physical anatomy. However, this cannot be the first point of intervention. Luke has several supportive figures in his life: his cousin, his school's gay-straight alliance, and his family members. Despite this, he remains depressed and has a genetic predisposition for anxiety. In this clinical vignette, maximizing his supports while aggressively treating Luke's depressive symptoms is the most appropriate initial course of action. For a supervisor and trainee, formulating the case in this manner is the most important component of the approach to any gender minority patient.

REFERENCES

1. Gordon AR, Meyer IH. Gender nonconformity as a target of prejudice, discrimination, and violence against LGB individuals. J LGBT Health Res 2007;3(3):55–71.
2. Lombardi EL, Wilchins RA, Priesing D, et al. Gender violence: transgender experiences with violence and discrimination. J Homosex 2001;42(1):89–101.
3. Factor RJ, Rothblum ED. A study of transgender adults and their non-transgender siblings on demographic characteristics, social support, and experiences of violence. J LGBT Health Res 2007;3(3):11–30.
4. The Harry Benjamin International Gender Dysphoria Association's standards of care for gender identity disorders. 6th version. World Professional Assiciation for Transgender Health. Available at: http://wpath.org/publications_standards.cfm. Published 2001. Accessed May 1, 2011.
5. Institutional programs and educational activities to address the needs of gay, lesbian, bisexual and transgender (GLBT) students and patients. Available at: https://www.aamc.org/download/157460/data/institutional_programs_and_educational_activities_to_address_th.pdf. Published 2007. Accessed May 1, 2011.
6. Kitts RL. Barriers to optimal care between physicians and lesbian, gay, bisexual, transgender, and questioning adolescent patients. J Homosex 2010;57(6):730–47.
7. Lena SM, Wiebe T, Ingram S, et al. Pediatricians' knowledge, perceptions, and attitudes towards providing health care for lesbian, gay, and bisexual adolescents. Ann R Coll Physicians Surg Can 2002;35(7):406–10.
8. Lena SM, Wiebe T, Ingram S, et al. Pediatric residents' knowledge, perceptions, and attitudes towards homosexually oriented youth. Ann R Coll Physicians Surg Can 2002;35(7):401–5.
9. Meyer-Bahlburg HF. From mental disorder to iatrogenic hypogonadism: dilemmas in conceptualizing gender identity variants as psychiatric conditions. Arch Sex Behav 2010;39(2):461–76.
10. American Psychiatric Association. Diagnostic and Statistical Manual of Mental Disorders. 4th edition. Washington, DC: American Psychiatric Association; 1994.
11. Wallien MS, Cohen-Kettenis PT. Psychosexual outcome of gender-dysphoric children. J Am Acad Child Adolesc Psychiatry 2008;47(12):1413–23.
12. Clements-Nolle K, Marx R, Guzman R, et al. HIV prevalence, risk behaviors, health care use, and mental health status of transgender persons: implications for public health intervention. Am J Public Health 2001;91(6):915–21.
13. Clements-Nolle K, Marx R, Katz M. Attempted suicide among transgender persons: the influence of gender-based discrimination and victimization. J Homosex 2006; 51(3):53–69.
14. Garofalo R, Deleon J, Osmer E, et al. Overlooked, misunderstood and at-risk: exploring the lives and HIV risk of ethnic minority male-to-female transgender youth. J Adolesc Health 2006;38(3):230–6.
15. Grossman AH, D'Augelli AR. Transgender youth and life-threatening behaviors. Suicide Life Threat Behav 2007;37(5):527–37.

16. Herbst JH, Jacobs ED, Finlayson TJ, et al. Estimating HIV prevalence and risk behaviors of transgender persons in the United States: a systematic review. AIDS Behav 2008;12(1):1–17.
17. Sausa LA, Keatley J, Operario D. Perceived risks and benefits of sex work among transgender women of color in San Francisco. Arch Sex Behav 2007;36(6):768–77.
18. Toomey RB, Ryan C, Diaz RM, et al. Gender-nonconforming lesbian, gay, bisexual, and transgender youth: school victimization and young adult psychosocial adjustment. Dev Psychol 2010;46(6):1580–9.
19. Wilson EC, Garofalo R, Harris DR, et al. Sexual risk taking among transgender male-to-female youths with different partner types. Am J Public Health 2010;100(8):1500–5.
20. Wilson EC, Garofalo R, Harris RD, et al. Transgender female youth and sex work: HIV risk and a comparison of life factors related to engagement in sex work. AIDS Behav 2009;13(5):902–13.
21. Pleak RR. Transgender persons. In: Ruiz P, Primm A, editors. Disparities in psychiatric care: clinical and cross-cultural perspectives. Philadelphia: Lipponcott Williams & Wilkins; 2010. p. 107–15.
22. Lambda Legal. When health care isn't caring: Lambda Legal's survey on discrimination against LGBT people and people living with HIV. Available at: http://data.lambdalegal.org/publications/downloads/whcic-report_when-health-care-isnt-caring.pdf. Published 2010. Accessed May 1, 2011.
23. University of California, San Francisco Center for LGBT Health & Equity. LGBT concerns in medical education: A tool for institutional self-assessment. Available at: http://lgbt.ucsf.edu/images/Institutional%20Self-Assessment%20AAMC.pdf. Published 2007. Accessed May 1, 2011.
24. Hoffman ND, Freeman K, Swann S. Healthcare preferences of lesbian, gay, bisexual, transgender and questioning youth. J Adolesc Health 2009;45(3):222–9.
25. The Endocrine Society. Endocrine treatment of transsexual persons: an Endocrine Society clinical practice guideline. Available at: http://www.endo-society.org/guidelines/final/upload/Endocrine-Treatment-of-Transsexual-Persons.pdf. Published 2009. Accessed May 1, 2011.
26. Association of American Medical Colleges. Cultural competence education. Available at: https://www.aamc.org/download/54338/data/culturalcomped.pdf. Published 2005. Accessed May 1, 2011.
27. Bussey K, Bandura A. Social cognitive theory of gender development and differentiation. Psychol Rev 1999;106(4):676–713.
28. Human Rights Campaign. Healthcare equality index. Available at: http://www.hrc.org/documents/HRC-Healthcare-Equality-Index-2010.pdf. Published 2010. Accessed May 1, 2011.

Index

Note: Page numbers of article titles are in **boldface** type.

United States Postal Service

Statement of Ownership, Management, and Circulation
(All Periodicals Publications Except Requestor Publications)

1. Publication Title	2. Publication Number	3. Filing Date
Child and Adolescent Psychiatric Clinics of North America	0 1 1 1 - 3 6 8 8	9/16/11

4. Issue Frequency	5. Number of Issues Published Annually	6. Annual Subscription Price
Jan, Apr, Jul, Oct	4	$275.00

7. Complete Mailing Address of Known Office of Publication (Not printer) (Street, city, county, state, and ZIP+4®)

Elsevier Inc.
360 Park Avenue South
New York, NY 10010-1710

Contact Person
Amy S. Beacham
Telephone (Include area code)
215-239-3687

8. Complete Mailing Address of Headquarters or General Business Office of Publisher (Not printer)

Elsevier Inc., 360 Park Avenue South, New York, NY 10010-1710

9. Full Names and Complete Mailing Addresses of Publisher, Editor, and Managing Editor (Do not leave blank)

Publisher (Name and complete mailing address)

Kim Murphy, Elsevier, Inc., 1600 John F. Kennedy Blvd. Suite 1800, Philadelphia, PA 19103-2899

Editor (Name and complete mailing address)

Sarah Barth, Elsevier, Inc., 1600 John F. Kennedy Blvd. Suite 1800, Philadelphia, PA 19103-2899

Managing Editor (Name and complete mailing address)

Sarah Barth, Elsevier, Inc., 1600 John F. Kennedy Blvd. Suite 1800, Philadelphia, PA 19103-2899

10. Owner (Do not leave blank. If the publication is owned by a corporation, give the name and address of the corporation immediately followed by the names and addresses of all stockholders owning or holding 1 percent or more of the total amount of stock. If not owned by a corporation, give the names and addresses of the individual owners. If owned by a partnership or other unincorporated firm, give its name and address as well as those of each individual owner. If the publication is published by a nonprofit organization, give its name and address.)

Full Name	Complete Mailing Address
Wholly owned subsidiary of	4520 East-West Highway
Reed/Elsevier, US holdings	Bethesda, MD 20814
N/A	

11. Known Bondholders, Mortgagees, and Other Security Holders Owning or Holding 1 Percent or More of Total Amount of Bonds, Mortgages, or Other Securities. If none, check box ☐ None

Full Name	Complete Mailing Address

12. Tax Status (For completion by nonprofit organizations authorized to mail at nonprofit rates) (Check one)
The purpose, function, and nonprofit status of this organization and the exempt status for federal income tax purposes:
☐ Has Not Changed During Preceding 12 Months
☐ Has Changed During Preceding 12 Months (Publisher must submit explanation of change with this statement)

PS Form 3526, September 2007 (Page 1 of 3 (Instructions Page 3)) PSN 7530-01-000-9931 PRIVACY NOTICE: See our Privacy policy in www.usps.com

---

13. Publication Title	14. Issue Date for Circulation Data Below
Child and Adolescent Psychiatric Clinics of North America	July 2011

15. Extent and Nature of Circulation		Average No. Copies Each Issue During Preceding 12 Months	No. Copies of Single Issue Published Nearest to Filing Date
a. Total Number of Copies (Net press run)		1147	1174
b. Paid Circulation (By Mail and Outside the Mail)	(1) Mailed Outside-County Paid Subscriptions Stated on PS Form 3541. (Include paid distribution above nominal rate, advertiser's proof copies, and exchange copies)	524	469
	(2) Mailed In-County Paid Subscriptions Stated on PS Form 3541 (Include paid distribution above nominal rate, advertiser's proof copies, and exchange copies)		
	(3) Paid Distribution Outside the Mails Including Sales Through Dealers and Carriers, Street Vendors, Counter Sales, and Other Paid Distribution Outside USPS®	86	88
	(4) Paid Distribution by Other Classes Mailed Through the USPS (e.g. First-Class Mail®)		
c. Total Paid Distribution (Sum of 15b (1), (2), (3), and (4))	►	610	557
d. Free or Nominal Rate Distribution (By Mail and Outside the Mail)	(1) Free or Nominal Rate Outside-County Copies Included on PS Form 3541	78	86
	(2) Free or Nominal Rate In-County Copies Included on PS Form 3541		
	(3) Free or Nominal Rate Copies Mailed at Other Classes Through the USPS (e.g. First-Class Mail)		
	(4) Free or Nominal Rate Distribution Outside the Mail (Carriers or other means)		
e. Total Free or Nominal Rate Distribution (Sum of 15d (1), (2), (3) and (4))	►	78	86
f. Total Distribution (Sum of 15c and 15e)	►	688	643
g. Copies not Distributed (See instructions to publishers #4 (page #3))	►	459	531
h. Total (Sum of 15f and g)	►	1147	1174
i. Percent Paid (15c divided by 15f times 100)	►	88.66%	86.63%

16. Publication of Statement of Ownership

☐ If the publication is a general publication, publication of this statement is required. Will be printed ☐ Publication not required
in the October 2011 issue of this publication.

17. Signature and Title of Editor, Publisher, Business Manager, or Owner

Amy S. Beacham Senior Inventory Distribution Coordinator

Date September 16, 2011

I certify that all information furnished on this form is true and complete. I understand that anyone who furnishes false or misleading information on this form or who omits material or information requested on the form may be subject to criminal sanctions (including fines and imprisonment) and/or civil sanctions (including civil penalties).

PS Form 3526, September 2007 (Page 2 of 3)

Printed and bound by CPI Group (UK) Ltd, Croydon, CR0 4YY

03/10/2024

01040455-0003